Bar Code Technology in Health Care:

A Tool for Enhancing Quality, Productivity and Cost Management

Karen M. Longe
Lisa B. Brenner

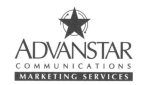

ADVANSTAR
COMMUNICATIONS
MARKETING SERVICES

Advanstar Communications, Inc.

Dedication

To Friendship

Printed in the United States of America

10 9 8 7 6 5 4 3 2 1

ISBN   0-929870-20-4

Library of Congress Catalog Card Number 93-71570

Published by ADVANSTAR Communications

ADVANSTAR Communications is a U.S. business information company that publishes magazines and journals, produces expositions and conferences, and provides a wide range of marketing services.

For additional information on any magazines or a complete catalog of ADVANSTAR Communications books, please write to ADVANSTAR Communications, Inc.; 7500 Old Oak Boulevard; Cleveland, OH 44130.

Table of Contents

Acknowledgments

The authors would like to acknowledge a number of individuals who gave their time and energy to help ensure the accuracy and readability of this publication.

Thanks to these individuals for reviewing chapters within their areas of expertise: Christina S. Barkan of Symbol Technologies, Inc.; Sue Chapin-Strike of The EDI Architect; Mark R. David of *Automatic I.D. News*; Susan Frankel formerly of the American Hospital Association; Clive P. Hohberger, Ph.D., of Zebra Technologies Corporation; Suzanna Hoppszallern of the American Hospital Association; Jane Lach of Deloitte Touche; and Kevin Sharp of Accurate Information.

We'd also like to thank the following individuals for their support and input: Yvonne Abdoo, Ph.D., RN, University of Michigan School of Nursing; George Armbruster of General Advanced Automation Technologies, Inc.; Craig K. Harmon of QED Systems; James McDonnell of J.E.M. Consulting; William Rose, Ph.D., of Rush-Presbyterian-St. Luke's Medical Center; Randy B. Scheib of Mediserve Information System; and Larry K. Shoup of Henry Ford Hospital.

Special thanks to Scott Cardais of Quad II and Mary E. Longe of Longe Life Libraries for their invaluable feedback on the manuscript. Our thanks and appreciation also goes to Paul E. Mehl for many years of guidance and support.

This publication would not have been possible without the support of John H. Kindsvater, Jr., Clive P. Hohberger, Ph.D., and W. Keith Everett of Zebra Technologies Corporation. We are also grateful for the input of countless people who use bar code technology in health care settings and were willing to share their experiences and insights with us.

Last, but not least, we'd also like to thank all those who helped make this publication a reality: Lori Fraser, Crista Zull and Paula Alward of Advanstar Communications; George Wong of The Design Office of George Wong; and Dave Crouch of Dave Crouch Graphics.

Introduction

Throughout the development of this book, we have been besieged by friends and colleagues wondering why we were going to the trouble to write a special book about bar code technology for health care. After all, publications and articles have been flooding the media for years about bar coding in different industries. There is certainly no shortage of resources explaining how bar code technology works. But as bar coding gains popularity and success in the health care industry, little has been written that demonstrates the effectiveness of bar coding specifically for health care applications. The purpose of this book, therefore, is to provide an overview of bar code technology in clear and simple language so that health care decision makers can make effective management decisions about using the technology within their institutions.

Why Bar Code Technology?

Before answering this question, it is important to understand that bar coding falls into a category of technologies known as **automatic data capture** or **automatic identification technologies**. The primary purpose of these technologies is to automate data entry so that basic information about people and/or products can be available through a computer more quickly and more accurately. With bar coding, information such as numbers, letters or graphic signals are encoded into bar codes — groupings of bars and spaces. These bars and spaces can then be read by a bar code scanner and converted into electronic symbols which provide automatic access to a database in a computer. It is important to understand that not all the information needed gets encoded into a bar code. The bar code contains an identification

The Bar Code Process

1. Label items.

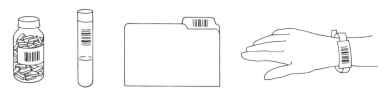

2. Scan the bar code label.

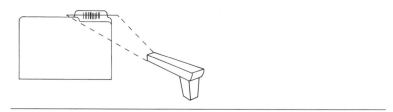

3. Access information on the computer.

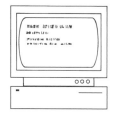

number, much as a license plate does. This number acts as key that opens up a database to the exact position containing all the information about the patient or product being identified.

Bar code technology is currently the most established automatic data capture technology with proven applications in health care in virtually every hospital department (see Chapter 1). Its adaptability to many different applications, ease of use, effectiveness and relative affordability make it a logical choice for improved data entry in health care settings. In fact, the technology is meeting with success in health care organizations worldwide. Implemented bar code applications from Australia, Canada, England, France, Germany, Italy, Japan, Korea, the

Netherlands, New Zealand, Norway, Portugal, Saudi Arabia, Singapore, Spain, Sweden and Switzerland as well as the United States were reviewed for this publication. Health care applications for bar coding can be found in almost every country in the world. Rest assured that your institution's first forays into bar coding will not require that the organization test the technology — bar coding is proven in health care.

While the authors are enthusiastic about the effectiveness of bar coding in health care, we must caution that the technology is not a panacea. Bar coding cannot solve all the information systems needs in health care because it only automates the front end, data capture. Bar coding also cannot repair a faulty manual system. If a poor, manual system is automated, health care executives cannot expect any real improvements. Those involved with the application must help evaluate a system before it is bar coded to achieve significant results (see Chapter 10).

What bar coding can do is a lot of what the health care industry is looking for: It can make the process of inputting information to a computerized system more accurate, timely, accessible, useful and cost effective. Ultimately, bar code technology provides better information for clinical and management decision making. For example:

Clinical Decision Making
- Bar coding test results speeds reports to clinicians for quicker clinical responsiveness.
- Bar coding drugs assures the availability of medication when and where it is needed.
- Bar coding medical histories makes critical, up-to-date information accessible throughout the hospital.

Management Decision Making
- Bar coding information provides timely, accurate data about resource utilization.
- Bar coding helps create objective quality measures based on real outcomes, which allows health care executives to negotiate more effectively with managed care providers.

Financial Decision Making

- Bar coding prevents lost charges resulting in better reimbursement.
- Bar coding eliminates duplication and waste, such as re-keying patient information in each department, which results in cost savings.
- Bar coding speeds claims processing resulting in improved cash flow.

Why Now?

Health care reform has moved to the forefront of our national agenda and will remain there for many years to come. Escalating health care costs are taxing everyone, including consumers, businesses and especially health care providers. Our system needs changes that work — a comprehensive set of options that will help direct us to:

- a basic level of health care accessible to everyone,
- decision making about which biotechnologies to pursue and which to put aside,
- better, less costly options for the provision of clinical care,
- more efficient administration and claims processing, and
- objective, measurable standards for evaluating the quality and results of patient care.

The Total Quality Management (TQM) and Continuous Quality Improvement (CQI) movements, in particular, have taken a strong hold in the health care industry. Most importantly, health care is an information industry. Information management is an integral part of every clinical and non-clinical action taken in the provision and delivery of health care. For all these reasons, now is the perfect time to evaluate any technology, old or new, that can improve information management and help make our health care system better.

The Golden Rule of Bar Coding

If there is one critical message for health care decision makers to understand about bar code technology it is what is referred to throughout this book as The Golden Rule of Bar Coding: Know Your Application. Bar coding can make a difference in simple processes (i.e. gas cylinder tracking) or complex processes (i.e. dispensing and administering drugs). By understanding what information is needed, by whom and why, you can build bar coding into an automated system — and a system which has a clear purpose. An application can also have implications for everything from the standards you follow (see Chapter 4) to the equipment you choose (see Chapter 5), to how you justify the implementation of bar coding (see Chapter 9) or, determining a need to integrate bar coding with other automatic data capture technologies (see Chapter 7).

Nothing demonstrates the effectiveness of bar code technology in health care better than existing applications. Throughout the book you'll find examples and case studies about bar code applications in health care. These examples come from a wide variety of hospitals worldwide — large and small, urban and rural, for-profit and not-for-profit, public, private and government owned — which have already implemented bar code applications. In some cases, the authors use specially designed examples to demonstrate how the technology's capabilities can satisfy emerging health care needs. No specific reference is made to hospital size or location in these cases.

Chapters in the book have been ordered to provide a logical progression for the reader in understanding bar coding and the decision making factors that health care executives must evaluate.

- *Chapter 1* introduces the fundamental concepts of bar code technology and explains the three primary functions of the technology in health care.
- *Chapter 2* summarizes a brief historical overview on the development of bar code technology.

- *Chapter 3* considers current trends and pressures in health care and how they might be improved with bar code technology.
- *Chapter 4* looks at how an institution can determine which bar code standards and symbologies to use for a given application.
- *Chapter 5* reviews bar code equipment considerations.
- *Chapter 6* discusses electronic data interchange, a complementary technology to bar coding, which provides the ability to exchange information electronically with organizations outside the institution.
- *Chapter 7* presents other automatic data capture technologies that can be used in conjunction with bar coding.
- *Chapter 8* demonstrates how all the concepts presented up to this point come together most effectively in health care by discussing the example of bar code technology and the emerging field of computer-based patient records.
- *Chapter 9* offers a systematic approach to creating quality measures and justifying health care investments in bar coding.
- *Chapter 10* explains the process health care institutions must undertake in order to implement bar code applications.

It is the authors' hope that this publication will motivate health care executives to implement bar coding in their own institutions. A simple application can be undertaken with limited expense and risk. Most importantly, a pilot bar code application is the best way to recognize the power and effectiveness of bar code technology.

Three Uses of Bar Code Technology: Tracking, Inventorying and Validating

As with any investment decision, health care executives must weigh the pros and cons of investing in bar code technology. Bar coding often reaps significant returns on investment in terms of finance, productivity, patient and employee satisfaction and quality. Experiences in other industries indicate that most organizations attain payback in two years, with many applications paying back in six to eighteen months. But change involves more than financial gain. What, then, are the benefits of automating health care systems with bar code technology? What can bar coding help you do that you aren't doing now?

Automatic data capture technologies, like bar coding, are tools for managing information better. Everything you do in a hospital involves information exchange — whether it's taking a medical history from a patient, reviewing x-rays or summarizing patient costs. Manual systems are slow, error prone and costly. In its simplest terms, the result of automating manual processes should be a system that allows you to find the information you need when you need it. This requires knowing:

- what information is needed,
- how, when and where to count or measure it,
- that information is accurate, and
- what constitutes meaningful output.

For bar code technology this translates into three primary functions: **tracking, inventorying** and **validating**. Whether you use one function or a combination of more than one, the benefits to health care organizations — in cost savings, improved productivity and quality — can be substantial.

Tracking

Anything and everything that can be represented as information can be tracked using bar code technology. Medical records, materials management and central service supplies, pharmaceuticals, laboratory tests and radiology files are common tracking applications in health care. Use is also increasing in areas such as admissions, respiratory therapy and blood transfusions. These technologies help speed the process of recording where and what an item is and assure greater accuracy.

Other vital applications for hospitals occur when patients and employees are tracked. As patients cross departments, they become information carriers. Tracking the patient ensures that procedures have occurred, responses are carefully monitored, all charges are properly allocated and much more. At the same time, employees across all departments effect change for patients. Nurses in particular serve as gatekeepers to the patient. Therefore, tracking the activities of these two groups can lead to invaluable management information.

One of the benefits of using bar code technology to track health care information is that it is multi-directional. Information can be tracked chronologically, in reverse chronological order, or in any direction you choose. For example, if a nurse discovers a defective IV bag when attempting to use it, bar coding can help track the item back through materials management and purchasing to the distributor and/or original manufacturer in order to obtain a refund.

You can also elect to track information in real time or batch time for different functions. Bar coding automatically records the time and date of every interaction when real time information is required. For instance, many hospitals use real time tracking to record the exact time a phlebotomist draws blood. On the other hand, there are many applications where batch time is adequate for data collection; information is scanned and collected over a period of time but loaded onto a computer in a batch at the end of a shift or a day. For example, batch tracking is typically used for recording items pulled from an exchange cart and allocated to each patient. Items are scanned as used, but recorded only at the end of a shift since the materials management department needs all the information at once to restock exchange carts and make inventory adjustments.

Here is a simple example of how bar code technology can help by tracking health care applications. Many hospitals lose $10,000 to $20,000 or more a year on charges for lost gas cylinder containers. Bar coding could completely eliminate these needless expenditures. A bar code could be attached to each gas cylinder container as it enters the hospital. Containers are scanned as they are dispersed throughout the hospital. In this way, staff can track missing containers so that they are returned to suppliers on time, eliminating additional charges.

The bottom line is that tracking systems help improve quality. More accurate tracking using bar code technology prevents errors, reduces lost charges and assures better quality throughout the system. A 400-bed hospital in New England was struggling with an inefficient medical records system. The costs for their high volume of medical record activity was escalating by $100,000 each year. At the same time:

- medical records were not available 60-70% of the time for same-day appointments,
- approximately 30 records a day for pre-scheduled appointments were not available when a patient arrived,
- it was taking an average of 20 minutes to locate lost records,
- an average of 18,000 records were located out of the department each week, and
- turnover rate for medical records personnel was 80%.

In some cases, physicians were hiding medical records to try to protect the confidentiality of patient information. The hospital implemented a bar code system for medical records tracking. As a result:

- operational costs for the medical records department decreased by $150,000 in the first year and $147,000 in the second year,
- on-time records deliveries increased to 91-94%, including same-day appointments,
- missing records for pre-scheduled appointments dropped to less than one per day,
- records located outside of the department decreased from 18,000 weekly to 7,500 weekly,
- the hospital reduced 11.5 medical records FTEs (full-time equivalent) over two years, and
- turnover rate in the department decreased to 40%.

Additionally, the department's capacity increased from handling 1,000-1,500 record requests weekly to implementing 3,500-4,000 weekly.

Many hospitals have staffs of FTEs hired exclusively for locating lost medical records.

Inventorying

Bar code technology has been successfully used for controlling inventories in countless industries. All businesses need to inventory what they have, how much of it they have, who has it, where it is, and if more is needed. In the complex domain of hospitals and other health care institutions, however, this involves levels of inventorying that touch every department. Every department maintains some supplies that need to be inventoried as part of the overall organizational effort. This includes everything from medical/surgical supplies, office supplies and linens to test tubes, x-ray film and pharmaceuticals. In some instances, such as with narcotics, additional inventory recording requirements may be needed. Effective management of inventories using bar code technology can help assure that the vital materials needed for patient care are available when and where you need them.

At the same time, bar coding allows health care organizations to monitor patterns of usage, reduce unnecessary inventory and shift to Just-In-Time inventorying methods. In one hospital, materials management wanted to reduce levels of unnecessary inventory on wards. Using bar code technology, they were able to monitor patterns of usage by individual units. Armed with real information, materials management staff began collaborating with nurses in each ward to create more realistic inventories. For example, if a particular unit was only using seven of one item a day but were keeping fifteen of the items on the floor, the two groups worked together to find a comfortable, lower figure. This saved the hospital inventory costs as well as strengthened communication between materials managers and nurses.

It is expected that the FDA will enforce a policy similar to the Medical Device Directives Act of Europe in the near future. The act requires tracking of medical devices to the patient in case of recalls.

Bar code technology can also help speed the process of reordering. Systems can be designed to automatically reorder when inventory reaches a predetermined level. One of the most advanced health care applications right now establishes a system where reordering is initiated for certain items directly from the nursing station. In a health care environment where time can cost lives, this capability can provide measurable savings as well as improve quality. A pharmacy's ability to reorder realistic inventories in a speedy fashion can help hospitals control cash flow while assuring that medications are always available.

In one large Midwestern hospital, the keypunch department was being eliminated in order to reduce costs. The pharmacy director convinced hospital executives to give him nine months to put a bar code system in place to replace the manual keypunch needed to keep the department operating. Bar code labels were applied to pharmacy shelving. A total of $45,000 was invested in implementing the system, including equipment purchase, software integration and staff training. The system saved the hospital $26,000 in one year and allowed for the redeployment of 1.5 FTEs. Payback for the system occurred in 1.7 years.

In one hospital, the implementation of a bar code system for inventory management reduced inventory reconciliation time from four or five days to four hours.

Validating

The validating function of bar coding can be an especially effective method for quality control in health care settings. These technologies help reduce errors and waste, provide a management check on productivity and construct the necessary documentation to meet Joint Commission on Accreditation of Healthcare Organizations (JCAHO) and/or insurance company requirements.

Validation assures that an action has taken place or that the item you want is the item in hand. Perhaps the single most important function of validation is to verify that the patient being treated is, in fact, the right patient. Nurses can use bar coding to confirm that the unit dose of a medication exactly matches the doctor's order before administering a drug, and to validate that they are giving the drug to the right patient. This process also immediately registers the drug application so that there is a record that the action took place. In this instance, bar coding assures that the medication is correct and is administered as needed.

How important is automated validation? A recent drug industry study points out how serious hospital drug errors can be. A survey of 361 hospital pharmacists and pharmacy directors asked about the causes and results of the institution's most recent drug errors. Here is how the cause of errors broke down:

- 48% of errors stemmed from giving the wrong drug.
- 34% of errors stemmed from giving the wrong dosage.
- 11% of errors stemmed from directing the drug through the wrong dispensing route.

And, what were the results?

- 39% of the time, the error was discovered before ingestion.
- 33% of the time, the patient suffered reversible side effects.
- 3% of the time, the patient had permanent side effects.
- 3% of the time, the patient died.

Automatic validation using bar code technology can help prevent these types of errors, reducing liability and improving the quality of care.

The validation function can also be used in non-patient care activities, such as equipment maintenance. By validating the steps a plant worker takes on biomedical equipment maintenance, health care institutions can automatically verify and record adherence with JCAHO standards. Validating the action helps prevent breakdowns and identifies the need for further repair before accidents occur. Finally, validating gives management a means of monitoring the worker's activity and productivity.

In Barcelona, Spain, one hospital is using a bar code system for tracking, inventorying and validating autologous and donor-directed blood. These blood donations must be carefully tested and separately inventoried. Additionally, the blood must be validated to ensure that the specimen at hand matches its intended patient. Bar coding provides a simple method for effectively accomplishing all three goals.

Integrating Functions

Many health care applications can take successful advantage of more than one function of bar code technology. Whether one or all three functions are used, bar coding is most effective when the system is integrated throughout the health care setting. Many clinical laboratories are already using bar code technology for tracking, validating and inventorying lab specimens. Below is a brief description of some of the real bar code applications being used with lab specimens.

Using bar coding, a doctor gives an order for a blood test. A phlebotomist is sent to the patient. Before drawing any blood, the phlebotomist scans the patient wristband to validate that it is the right patient. The phlebotomist is identified by scanning the employee's identification badge. The bar code system also automatically records real time for the blood draw. Immediately after drawing blood, the phlebotomist bar code labels the specimen. The phlebotomist drops the needle into a bar coded sharps container. The specimen is taken to the laboratory, the bar code label is scanned and the information is downloaded into the system.

In the laboratory, the specimen is scanned upon entry. Specimens are placed on a lab analyzer that has built-in bar code capabilities. The analyzer automatically reads the bar code, registers the information about the desired test(s), conducts the appropriate tests and outputs a test report. Systems can even be devised so that physicians can automatically check the status of the specimen on a computer.

One hospital is using bar coding to inventory specimens while they are retained in case of retesting. Using a bar code menu, each specimen is assigned a location in a refrigeration unit. When the specimen is called for retesting, a simple scan identifies the location and validates that the specimen at hand is the one desired. Timely purging of unneeded samples is also simplified through the bar coded inventory of specimens. With the bar code system, the hospital has reduced searches for specimens from an average of ten minutes to seconds, saving more than six hours per day.

By the way, bar coding is an excellent method for complying to regulations for sharps container disposal. The proper handling and disposal of sharps containers for health care organizations is strictly mandated by the Occupational Safety and Health Administration (OSHA) and the Environmental Protection Agency (EPA). Institutions are required to follow explicit procedures for handling the containers within the institution, contract with specially licensed medical waste haulers and deliver properly completed manifests with each shipment. Bar coding the system can help reduce liability and quickly document compliance to regulations. If each container is bar coded, it can be scanned at regular intervals to confirm the container's location in the hospital, its status (empty or full) and every action taken with the container (i.e. moving it, replacing it, preparing it for return shipment). Automatic reports can also be generated using the bar coded system.

A Bar Coded Day in the Life of One Patient

While many health care applications happen behind the scenes and are invisible to patients, most patients perceive the bar-coded functions they do see as beneficial because they are easy and quick. Let's take a look at one example showing how a patient sees bar code applications during a hospital stay — in this case, a women being admitted to the hospital to deliver a baby.

• *In admissions, the woman is given a wristband containing her bar coded patient identification number. Her chart is bar coded with the same number at the same time.*

- *In the labor room, nurses record the woman's vital signs with a bar code scanner.*
- *A nurse draws blood for standard blood work. The tube is bar coded for immediate scanning. The sample is sent to the lab.*
- *In the laboratory, a lab analyzer reads the information directly off the bar code, conducts the test and provides a test report without any human intervention.*
- *At the same time, a nurse uses bar coding to schedule the delivery room, schedule a crib, order sterilized surgical equipment and send swaddling and diapers to the nursery.*
- *After delivery, the baby's wrist and ankle are banded for tracking and recording all future information on its own chart. The father's wrist is also banded to track visits.*
- *The doctor orders medication for the patient. A nurse scans a code for the specific medication, which is automatically conveyed to the pharmacy.*
- *In the pharmacy, bar coding is used to dispense the medication. The pharmacist scans the unit dose and the patient number to verify the correct dispensing and automatically adjust the inventory. Back in the patient care unit, the nurse scans the medication to verify that the medication, patient and dosage are correct and to record the administration of the drug.*
- *Mother and baby are wheeled to discharge in a wheelchair that was scheduled through a bar coded porter system.*

• *At check-out time, a bill for all up-to-the-minute chargeable expenses is automatically prepared from the information recorded during the woman's and baby's stay through bar code technology.*

Health Care Applications

Health care applications using bar code technology began approximately 20 years ago for blood banking and inventorying. Today, bar code applications can be found for most hospital departments and in most health care settings. To help you understand the potential these technologies offer, below is a departmental listing of current bar code applications in hospitals. These examples were culled from real hospitals of all sizes.

Admissions
• Patient wristbands
• Charts

Asset/Property Management
• Preventive equipment maintenance
• Equipment inventorying
• Fixed asset management
• Capital asset tracking

Clinical Laboratory/Blood Bank
• Specimen labeling and tracking
• Test reporting

Clinical Laboratory/Blood Bank *continued*
• Monitor reagents on automated chemistry analyzers
• Blood and blood products inventorying
• Blood transfusion documentation
• Tracking blood donors
• Patient file tracking

Library
• Patron identification cards
• Book check-out and return
• Inventorying books and journals

Management Engineering
- Data collection
- Time study work samplings to generate statistical reports

Materials Management/ Central Supply/Purchasing
- Inventory control and warehousing
- Shelf location labels for restocking
- Vendor order entry
- Inventory transactions
- Maintaining par levels
- Suture inventory control
- Exchange cart inventory control and distribution
- Patient charge reconciliation and recovery
- Storeroom supplies
- Gas cylinder tracking
- Inventorying forms
- Patient rental equipment
- Scheduling operating rooms and services
- Linen inventory and distribution
- Warehouse location recording
- Cycle counting/annual inventories
- Order entry for dietary supplies
- Annual equipment inventories

Medical Records
- Record requests
- Record tracking and control (inpatient and outpatient)
- Deficiency management
- Productivity reporting
- Record volume

Nursing
- Nursing acuity system
- Bedside care
- Nursing patient classification system

Personnel
- Personnel document tracking
- Identification badges
- Time and attendance records
- Security access to parking and building structures

Pharmacy
- Order entry
- Daily and annual inventorying
- Billing
- Charge capture
- Inventory control
- Refilling prescriptions
- Pharmacy stock management
- Reordering from wholesalers and manufacturers
- Outpatient prescriptions and refills
- Pharmacy labels
- Narcotics control

Radiology

- Film file tracking
- Record procedures
- Report entry
- Patient registration
- Patient status
- Results reporting
- Scheduling
- Exam transactions
- Film quality control
- Charge capture and billing

Respiratory Therapy

- Charge determination
- Assessment documentation
- Patient scheduling
- Staff scheduling
- Treatment orders
- Documentation of provided therapies
- Treatment results
- Equipment tracking and maintenance
- Charge capture
- Quality assurance data collection

Benefits of Using Bar Code Technology

Different applications yield different benefits when using bar coding, yet opportunities for measurable, profitable and satisfying improvements abound. For health care organizations, bar code technology can have particular value in improving quality care, increasing patient satisfaction, capturing charges and making important information available more quickly.

An innovative British dentist has streamlined the time and cost of resource management using a bar code system. The dentist sees approximately 1,000 patients a month. By creating a menu-driven bar code system for managing patient information and patient communications, the dentist was able to improve resource management, increase throughput and free staff for clinical support duties.

Chapter 9 describes how to justify the expenditure for investing in bar coding. In general, however, there is much for health care institutions to gain from using these technologies.

Cost Savings

- Health care organizations can better manage assets and control cash flow with the information that is readily available using bar code technology.
- Reductions in errors and waste can be a direct result of automating a manual system.
- Bar coding provides immediate information about utilization so that the cost efficiency of each department and procedure can be better managed.
- Bar coding can help keep equipment costs down.
- Labor cost reductions result from bar coding efficiencies.
- Bar coding systematizes and assures that lost charges are captured.
- Malpractice costs are reduced because of improved documentation.

Efficiency

- Automated systems can be quicker and more accurate than manual ones.
- Bar coding offers the ability to provide greater detail to the extent you need it when and where you need it.
- Bar coding can assure availability of records, supplies, pharmaceuticals, equipment, operating rooms — even nurses.
- More than one person can use the system at one time.
- Bar code technology helps standardize and organize procedures.
- Bar coding makes information accessible and communicable more quickly.
- JCAHO compliance is quicker and easier to document.

Patient Satisfaction

- Patient satisfaction is increased as staff is more responsive, less error prone and offers more attention in giving care.

Productivity

- Managing productivity and identifying staff problems can be augmented with information from bar code systems.
- Bar coding can help alleviate labor shortages. Nurses alone are said to spend 30% of their time on documentation.
- Automated systems promote coordination and teamwork both in and between departments. This often reduces duplicated efforts.
- By monitoring usage patterns, health care institutions can improve resource utilization using bar code technology.
- Management obtains more accurate, detailed information on which to base decisions when bar code applications are in place.
- Bar coding can improve equipment safety and availability by implementing regular maintenance activities.
- Bar coding helps reduce overtime and its concomitant costs.

Quality

- Because staff are not tied to documentation, their professional satisfaction increases, stress is reduced and they can spend more time where it matters — providing quality care.
- Automated systems of checks and balances using bar code technology help health care organizations maintain quality control in everything from medication administration to equipment maintenance.
- Automatic verification through the validating function of bar code technology can help prevent errors before they occur. This supports risk management efforts and may even help reduce liability.
- Greater efficiency in scheduling and delivery of care gives patients a better sense about the quality of care they are receiving.

Summary

Bar coding is a tool for making information management quicker, easier and more accurate. Bar coding serves three major functions: tracking, inventorying and validating information exchanges. In general, bar code technology improves information accuracy, speeds information availability, and frees staff in health care settings to uphold their primary mission — providing quality care.

An Historical Overview of Bar Code Technology

Like many technologies, bar coding had a slow start. The full potential of bar code technology was not fully realized until it became economically viable. The earliest suggested bar code application can be traced back to the retail food industry in the 1930s. But it wasn't until the 1950s that both the retail food industry and railroad industry pursued serious developments for bar code symbologies and standards. By the 1970s, bar code technology was a staple of manufacturing, primarily for purchasing and inventorying functions. It was under the auspices of these manufacturing-related applications that bar coding entered the health care arena. In the 1980s, bar code technology was pervasive enough for the health care industry to approve its own symbology and applications standards. This chapter provides an historical overview of the development of bar code technology.

Supermarket Ideas and Inventions

Antecedents for bar code technology date back to the 1930s when Wallace Flint, the son of a Piggly Wiggly store owner in Massachusetts, prepared a master's thesis at Harvard Graduate School of Business about automating supermarket checkout counters. The project proposed using flow racks and punch cards to automatically dispense products to customers and calculate charges. After graduating, he and a team of colleagues offered the idea to food chains across the country. However, extremely low labor costs and high capital investment requirements made the idea economically impractical. While the idea was not lost, little progress was made again on bar code technology until the late 1940s, when supermarket labor costs were no longer so low and the industry was seeking ways to improve productivity.

By the late 1940s, the National Association of Food Chains was studying a number of inventions for automating grocery store checkout. The first machine readable code, called the **Bulls Eye Code**, was patented in 1949 by Joseph Woodland and Bernard Silver. As you can see in Figure 1-1, the circular code was, in fact, bars and spaces organized in a curve. Many inventors tried their hand at other types of bar codes in the 1950s and 1960s. Finally, from 1968 to 1972, the retail food industry conducted a pilot study using the Bulls Eye Code for supermarket checkout. In addition to speeding grocery store checkout, the test provided store owners with significant, new information for cost/benefit analyses. As a result, the system was refined and an ad hoc committee in the retail food industry was established to look at the possibility of universal product coding.

Figure 1-1 – Bull's Eye Code

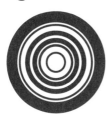

In April 1973, the U.S. Supermarket Ad Hoc Committee on Universal Product Coding approved the **Universal Product Code** (U.P.C.), the bar code symbology that still prevails in many retail industries. European countries followed suit with the adoption of the European Article Numbering (EAN) system in 1976, now called EAN International. In June 1974, the first scanning system was installed at a Marsh's Store in Troy, Ohio. By 1980, more than 90% of all grocery store items carried the U.P.C. code. And, by December 1985, more than 12,000 grocery stores were equipped with scanner checkout systems. In the short span of a decade, the grocery industry had been revolutionized using bar code technology.

Railroads Spearhead Other Applications

Service and manufacturing interests in bar coding began with the railroad industry in the 1950s. Their first breakthrough came relatively quickly: in 1962, E. F. Brinker filed a patent for an optical bar code system that attached to the side of railroad cars. The technology used retroreflective blue, red and white bars, which could be read from a distance as a railroad car passed a scanner placed by the track. The North American Railroad Industry adopted the bar code system in 1967 based on the understanding that it would be a low maintenance technology. By 1974, more than $2 million had been spent to label 95% of freight cars in the country. That same year, the system was abandoned due to significant maintenance (labels had to be cleaned regularly so that they could be read), training and equipment costs.

Sample Codes

U.P.C.

Code 49

Code 39

PDF417

Meanwhile, bar code symbologies were being developed for worldwide applications. In 1971, the first European symbology was introduced by the Plessey Company. This numeric code was originally designed for the U.K. Ministry of Defense to keep track of files, but the Ministry never implemented the system. However, the technology was not wasted — the Plessey Code is still widely used for library applications around the globe. In 1972, Codabar, the only symbology at the time that incorporated a method for checking accuracy, was quickly accepted for blood banking, library and air parcel industries. Codabar is the symbology used by Federal Express. In 1974, Code 39, the first symbology that used both numbers and letters (alphanumeric), was created.

With the adoption of the U.P.C. code in the retail industry, bar code uses expanded while most industries recognized the need for greater standardization. In 1982, the U.S. Department of Defense mandated that suppliers use bar codes on all incoming packaging. This affected nearly 50,000 government suppliers and firmly established Code 39 as the industrial applications code.

The remainder of the 1980s were marked by a proliferation of applications across all industries and the acceptance of industry standards. Code 128 was introduced by Computer Identics in 1981. In 1983, American National Standards Institute (ANSI) approved standards for Code 39, Interleaved 2 of 5 and Codabar. In 1984, the U.P.C. Shipping Container symbol (Interleaved 2 of 5) was adopted. The automotive industry selected Code 39 as its industry standard for shipping container labels. Also in 1984, the Health Industry Bar Code Council adopted the Code 39 symbology and its first standard for suppliers, followed in 1985 by a standard for providers.

After 1985, each year brought new and expanding capabilities to bar code technology. In the late 1980s, the first **two-dimensional** or **stacked** bar codes were introduced (Code 49 and Code 16K). These symbologies look like a checkerboard and offer a way of encoding data in a smaller space. The two symbologies were developed with health care and electronics applications in mind. The most recent technological breakthrough in bar coding has been the **matrix** bar code, such as PDF417 and DataMatrix. The storage capacity of these bar code symbologies is so vast that the entire Gettysburg Address can be encoded in approximately a two-inch square symbol.

Today, bar code technology represents $3.5 billion in business for hardware and software manufacturers, distributors and system integrators. Current projections indicate that the industry is growing at about 20% a year. Bar coding is used in almost every industry imaginable. For example, tiny bar codes were used in a research study to track bees going in and out of hives. Munitions management for Desert Storm was augmented by bar code technology. Most movie theaters use bar code technology to open curtains, start the projector and change reels. It is no exaggeration to say that, in one way or another, bar code technology touches on almost every aspect of daily living around the world.

Trends in Health Care: Where Does Bar Code Technology Fit?

The burden of escalating costs, lower margins and fierce competition are threatening the very existence of health care providers today. While reforms are needed on all levels of health care delivery (i.e. clinical, management, finance and administration), one thing is certain — our nation's health care system can no longer afford waste and ineffectual operations. Some experts project that waste, fraud and duplication add up to $58 million in excessive administrative costs for the nation's health system. Eliminating waste and streamlining operations throughout health care institutions are becoming mandatory steps for survival.

In order to reduce the costs and assure a high level of quality care in our nation's health care system, we must have accurate, reliable and available information. Information systems will become the vital link for capturing, sharing, and managing the information health care decision makers will need. Because of its speed, accuracy and ease of use, bar coding, in particular, can serve a crucial role in assuring the accessibility of correct data. This chapter looks at the potential link between trends in health care and uses for bar coding. The effectiveness of bar code technology is analyzed in the context of four critical health care reform issues.

Why Bar Coding?

While bar code technology is by no means a panacea for health care reform, its capabilities are ideal for responding to many of the problems facing our health care system. Health care is an information intensive industry. Hospitals, physicians, managed care providers, insurance companies, employers, the government and consumers are demanding access to a myriad of vital information about costs and quality of care. Bar coding is an affordable tool that can be used to capture all pertinent health care information — from medical histories and patient charts to insurance eligibility and claims processing — and make it accessible to those who need it when they need it.

Information systems improvements and bar code technology will enhance health care reforms in four pivotal areas: quality of care, regionalization, cost management and claims processing.

Quality of Care

The American health care system is said to provide the highest quality care in the world. But what constitutes "quality care"? How good must care be in order to qualify as "quality"? Where is the dividing line between acceptable and non-acceptable quality of care? As our nation curtails health expenditures, how can we be sure that articulated standards for "quality care" are maintained?

In attempting to define levels of care that are acceptable to patients, employers, the government and third-party payers, health care providers will have to find methods for measuring and documenting quality. Total Quality Management, Continuous Quality Improvement and information systems will be the glue that holds these measurement systems together. Accessible, speedy and accurate systems must be in place so that information can be captured at every juncture in the health delivery process for evaluation and comparison. This will be the basis for determining whether a patient received an acceptable level of quality care.

Creating quality measures requires establishing a whole new set of information that hasn't existed in the past. Bar code technology can make this type of data capture efficient and dependable. A growing trend among health care providers is the development of **outcomes measurements** — information derived from tracking real outcomes to specific diagnoses, procedures and treatments. This information is also being used to identify wasteful or ineffective processes and caregivers and to establish **clinical practice parameters** or **protocols** — clinical guidelines for treating a particular diagnosis based on statistical review of real cases, preferably in the same health care setting. Outcomes measurements offer continuous, real information on which key players (hospitals, managed care providers, other health care providers, physicians, insurance companies, employers and the government) in the health care system can base quality of care and cost containment choices. The ultimate result of using outcomes measurements should be better delivery of care at the same time that costs are managed throughout the health care system.

Figure 3-1 – Driving Costs (1980–89)

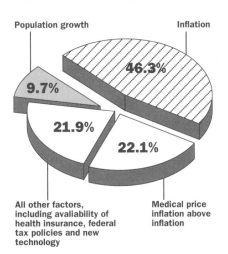

SOURCE: Health Care Financing Administration. National Journal, 2/15/92.

Bar coding can have an even more direct impact on quality of care. The speed and accuracy of bar code technology assures patients of receiving the right care faster, such as having medical records available when and where they are needed. The technology also reduces the time caregivers (nurses, doctors and technicians) spend on paperwork, allowing them to spend more time in direct contact with patients and, at the same time, improving documentation.

Regionalization

Regionalization is the byword for the future of health care delivery systems. Too many competing health care providers are creating excessive and unnecessary waste and duplication. For the past few years, many health care reformists recommended a move toward managed competition, a system in which providers compete according to general rules set by the government and under government scrutiny. More recently, health care experts have introduced a new concept called managed collaboration, a system where providers work together under a general set of government rules and government scrutiny. As a result, the health care system is expected to reshape itself into regional delivery systems. Regional systems will emerge, connecting hospitals, outpatient and ambulatory care clinics and physicians into an integrated system for care. This will allow institutions to save costs by sharing expenditures for biomedical equipment and information systems, streamlining administration, reducing duplication and much more.

As regional delivery systems develop, information will have to be shared in a timely manner among hospitals, physicians, outpatient centers, ambulatory care clinics, managed care providers, insurance companies and other health care agencies. Automating clinical information in the form of electronic medical records is a hot topic among technology providers and health care decision makers alike. Sharing common patient information can speed

Figure 3-2 – Paying the Health Care Bill

(1980 – Total: $250.2 billion)

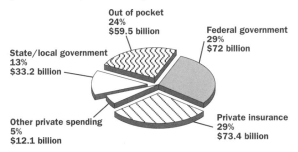

Out of pocket
24%
$59.5 billion

Federal government
29%
$72 billion

State/local government
13%
$33.2 billion

Private insurance
29%
$73.4 billion

Other private spending
5%
$12.1 billion

(1990 – Total: $666.2 billion)

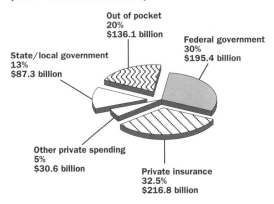

Out of pocket
20%
$136.1 billion

Federal government
30%
$195.4 billion

State/local government
13%
$87.3 billion

Private insurance
32.5%
$216.8 billion

Other private spending
5%
$30.6 billion

SOURCE: Health Care Financing Administration. National Journal, 2/15/92.

the process of diagnosis and treatment, reduce wasteful administrative practices and improve billing and reimbursement accuracy and efficiencies. Shared information also allows health care decision makers to aggregate and compare information collected throughout the system. Flexible information systems must be put in place that permit quick and easy information exchange and quick access to off-line, archived information. Bar code technology combined with electronic data interchange (EDI) [see Chapter 6] will become dominant, formidable tools for efficient information exchange.

Cost Management

While one-time savings throughout the health care system can make a significant dent toward reducing expenditures, the cost problems facing our health care system cannot be resolved until the ongoing costs for delivering care are brought down. No doubt the current trend in government caps on health care expenditures will continue while more emphasis will be placed on reducing administrative waste and fraud in the health care system. The federal government will also concentrate efforts on redefining financial responsibility for the medical costs and how costs for the uninsured and underinsured will be shared among the key players. Despite these efforts, it is the ongoing, incremental improvements throughout the health care delivery system that will have the most impact on controlling costs.

Information systems that help improve cost management will offer health care decision makers information to avoid costly errors, determine trends for cost efficiencies and savings and track the return-on-investment for expenditures. Bar coding, in particular, can help health care providers reduce the incremental costs associated with day-to-day operations. Bar code technology guarantees speedier and more accurate data capture for better and more flexible financial management information. Additionally, time saved using bar coding instead of manual systems can improve resource management and staff productivity.

Another important player in the demand for better management of health care costs is employers. Because employers remain one of the major health care payers, expect them to continue exerting their buying power to ensure quality of care and lower costs for services provided to their employees. Employers will demand results from hospitals and managed care providers in the form of outcomes measurements and proven cost savings. Improved information systems that use bar code technology for data capture can help ensure that employers get the results they demand without taxing providers.

Claims Processing

One area where incremental savings can make a big difference is claims processing. Our nation processes about 4 billion claims each year. The Congressional Budget Office estimated that a shift from more than 1,500 health care plans to a single plan in 1989 would have saved the country $58 billion in reduced administrative costs for insurers, doctors and hospitals. As a country, we can no longer afford such high levels of administrative waste. Whether a single plan is accepted or not, recommendations have been made to shift to electronic claims processing using a single claim form for all payers. By combining electronic data interchange with bar coding, electronic claims processing can replace the bulk of the current paper system, creating significant time, productivity and cost savings. Efforts are already underway to devise computer standards and protocols for electronic claims processing.

Summary

Dramatic reform in the nation's health care system is needed in order to reduce costs, assure quality and provide access to health care for all people. The health care environment will take on a new shape as fewer providers work in regional systems for delivering and financing care. Outcomes measurements and clinical practice protocols will change the way providers and payers evaluate the quality and cost of care. Measuring quality, reducing costs, streamlining administration, building greater efficiencies, heightening productivity and making information accessible to multiple users at various sites will all be accelerated with the help of improved information systems and automatic data capture technologies. Bar code technology is particularly appropriate for providing the flexibility, speed and accuracy needed for data capture in health care.

Other Motivating Factors

- *The Health Care Financing Administration (HCFA), projects that the country will spend $1.6 trillion for health care in the year 2000 which will be 16.4% of the Gross National Product and one of the largest categories in our nation's budget.*
- *The U.S. outspends every other nation in health care expenditures.*
- *According to the Health Care Financing Administration, Medicare Part A, the trust fund for the federal hospital insurance program, will be exhausted by the year 2005.*
- *Between 33 and 38 million people have neither private nor public insurance. Another 30 million people have coverage that experts regard as inadequate.*
- *Medical bills were the leading cause of personal bankruptcy in 1992.*
- *Ford Motor Company reported that 20% of all payroll costs in 1992 went to health care.*
- *Throughout the automotive industry, these health care costs add $500 to $700 per car.*

Standards and Symbologies: The Language of Bar Code Technology

Standards and symbologies: two words in bar coding that are both deceptively simple and deceptively complex. It is tempting to delegate responsibility for knowing the meaning behind these terms to technical advisors and information systems specialists. However, a basic understanding of the technology behind bar coding is key to getting the best results from your system. Therefore, it is important to have a fundamental understanding of the underlying concepts. In this chapter, we will review the process that starts with your proposed application and leads to the appropriate standards and bar code symbology. The important concepts involved in bar code standards and symbologies will also be explained in non-technical language.

What Information Is Needed?

The best place to start evaluating standards and symbologies is with the application itself. Within specific applications, each item to which a bar code will be attached must be analyzed in order to determine what information needs to be encoded. For example, tracking a medication requires information that identifies the product (i.e. a product number and a manufacturer's code) and possibly the unit dose. On a patient wristband, information needs to be encoded so that the patient can be identified. Remember, most of the bar codes used in health care today do not encode all information about a person or thing. They only contain one basic identification number which acts like a license plate number.

When the symbol (number) is scanned, it provides a link to a computer and offers access to a database containing all the information detail you seek.

Fortunately, there is no need to create a special numbering system for bar code technology. Most numbering systems, such as National Drug Codes for drug products, social security numbers for patients or any other patient numbering system you may use, can be encoded in a bar code. Once you determine what information needs to be encoded, industry standards for applications and labeling provide guidelines for the format and structure of the information within the bar code.

Open and Closed Systems

Another important concept to understand in preparing for bar coding is determining whether your applications will be in an open or closed system. An **open system** is characterized by the ability to encode a bar code label in one place and decode it at another. The person using the bar code may not be identifiable by the labeler, so no special equipment or knowledge other than common knowledge encoded in the symbology and standards can apply. For example, a pharmaceutical product bar coded by the manufacturer can be read in any health care setting when the system is open. A **closed system** occurs in a completely manageable environment, where a central authority defines how the equipment encodes, decodes and processes the data. For example, in the case of a clinical trial, a closed system may be appropriate because of the limited number of people involved and the importance of maintaining strict data integrity.

In general, however, hospitals are open systems. Patients, employees, records and resources move from department to department. Bar coded supplies, which need to be scanned in many departments, come to the hospital from external manufacturers and distributors. Additionally, under new health care reforms, patient information — the most important data a hospital will bar code — will be shared more often among physician offices, laboratories and other outpatient and ambulatory care settings outside the hospital's bar code system. Any bar coded information and/or products coming into your system from the outside or going from your system outside (i.e. organ transplant information) won't necessarily be compatible — or usable — if your system is closed. Be sure to recognize all possible applications before limiting your organization to a closed system.

Application Standards

Because health care institutions are for the most part open systems, these organizations need to abide by application standards for bar coding. Application standards have been established in most industries so that a bar code symbol created anywhere (such as a pharmaceutical manufacturer or distributor) can be scanned and decoded anywhere (such as a health care institution). Bar code standards should not be confused with the typical "standards" encountered by health care organizations (i.e. JCAHO standards). Bar code standards exist solely to facilitate communication. What they actually "standardize" is the format for communications. The consistency that results from application standards guarantees communication between product manufacturers, distributors and end-users, assures that bar codes are readable worldwide and helps streamline equipment choices for all parties.

In health care, application standards become even more vital when dealing with patient applications. Using application standards, patients not only can be tracked efficiently through every department in a hospital, but timely clinical information can be retrieved or communicated to doctors' offices, independent laboratories and other outpatient and ambulatory care centers. This capability will help health care providers even more as reform moves in the direction of regionalization.

Adhering to application standards for the health care

industry is essential and can help you accrue a number of significant benefits. These include:

- assuring easier communications between departments,
- improving communication between medical product suppliers and health care institutions,
- increasing efficiency in handling items,
- increasing productivity in processing bar coded items,
- guaranteeing information accessibility for all bar code users and equipment,
- saving costs in equipment purchase, communications and handling, and
- preventing costly equipment selection errors.

Health care standards for bar code technology are developed by the Health Industry Business Communications Council (HIBCC). This organization is a coalition of five major health care associations: the American Hospital Association (AHA), Health Industry Distributors Association (HIDA), Health Industry Manufacturers Association (HIMA), National Wholesale Druggists' Association (NWDA) and the Pharmaceutical Manufacturers Association (PMA). The standards developed by the HIBCC describe the data that is to be encoded and specify which symbology is recommended for health care applications. The European Health Industry Business Communications Council (EHIBCC), the European counterpart to the HIBCC, promotes the same standards. When your technical team members reach the symbology selection stage, make sure they get copies of the existing standards and use them instead of spending time trying to develop their own.

Requirements for Labeling Bar Code Products

In 1984, the HIBCC approved the Supplier Labeling Standard, which prescribes specific requirements for healthcare suppliers to bar code their products. The standard suggests, but does not mandate, that the supplier (either a manufacturer or distributor) use a primary code and offers an optional secondary code. The primary code is made up of the Labeler Identification Code (LIC; a number purchased by the supplier from HIBCC), the supplier's product number and a unit of measure. That LIC is maintained by HIBCC to make sure that the same manufacturer always uses that same identification number. The optional secondary label — used in conjunction with the primary label — includes an expiration date and a lot, batch or serial number.

Here is an example of a Code 39 bar code symbol using the Supplier Labeling Standard:

Figure 4-1

Stipulation of what information is included, its order and format, is what is known as the data structure. The **data structure** for the Supplier Labeling Standard is demonstrated in Figure 4-1. The asterisks are start and stop characters required by the symbology. The "+" is a data identifier indicating a health industry bar code. H123 is the Labeler Identification Code, and 798432 is the product number. The next number, "1", is the unit of measure. The "C" at the end is a check character used to ensure additional data security. With this labeling standard, health care suppliers worldwide can produce bar codes that contain information encoded in this manner.

HIBCC quickly followed the Supplier Labeling Standard with the Provider Application Standard in 1985. This standard was devised for patient care bar code applications in all major functional areas of health care organizations. Special characters, known as **data identifiers** or **flag characters**, identify the type of data that follows. In health care, two data identifiers are used in tandem so that hospitals can determine where the information is coming from (i.e. a patient wristband versus a patient record) and what the information is (i.e. patient identification).

Figure 4-2

Figure 4-3

Figures 4-2 and 4-3 are examples of bar codes following the HIBC Provider Applications Standard. The bar codes use asterisks at the beginning and end as "start" and "stop" characters. The "A" in Figure 4-2 indicates a patient and the "C" means Patient Identification, indicating that a patient identification number will follow. In Figure 4-3, the "B" indicates a patient care record and the "C", once again, indicates that Patient Identification follows. In both figures, the patient identification number is 493674. The last character is a check character to ensure data security. When the bar code is scanned, the data identifiers tell the computer where the information was located (on a patient wristband in the first figure and on a patient record in the second figure) and what the information is (patient identification). This is particularly important when positive patient identification is critical, such as when a patient receives a blood transfusion.

A review of application and labeling standards for the health care industry provides the format for organizing information within a bar code. Now the only remaining step is choosing a symbology.

Health Industry Standards

Within the health care industry, certain groups have taken the HIBC standards a step further to create greater specificity about data structures and symbologies used for their particular interests.

- *The National Wholesale Druggists' Association (NWDA) published a position paper on "Numerical and Automatic Identification of Drug Products in Distribution and Patient Care." The paper reinforces the use of HIBC standards and adds guidelines for labeling packaging at all levels (i.e. shipping cases, intermediate packaging, and large and small unit-of-use packages).*

- *The Health Industry Distributors Association (HIDA) developed a position paper about "Bar Coding of Medical/ Surgical Products in Distribution and Patient Care."*

- *ASTM (American Society for Testing and Materials) extended the HIBC Provider Applications Standard with its own guidelines, "Standard Specification for Use of Bar Codes on Specimen Tubes in the Clinical Laboratory." This standard recommends the use of Code 39 or Code 128 in the laboratory and reinforces the data structure offered by the HIBCC. It also describes label orientation and placement and symbol size to facilitate the effective use of bar code readers in clinical laboratory analyzers.*

> *• A worldwide standard for bar code labeling of blood and blood products is currently being developed by the International Society for Blood Transfusion (ISBT) in cooperation with the HIBCC. The standard, "ISBT 128 Bar Code Symbology and Application Specifications for Blood and Blood Products Labeling," will use Code 128 after a migration from Codabar — the previously used symbology. PDF417 is also being studied.*

What Is a Symbology?

Symbology is the language of bar coding. In a symbology, information is encoded using groupings of light spaces and dark bars. By varying the width and patterns of the bars and spaces, a symbol is created which represents a number, letter, punctuation or graphic (i.e. 4, A, $, %). Some symbologies encode only numbers, others encode numbers and letters (alphanumeric). The sample bar codes for different symbologies on page 40 show you how different these arrangements can be.

There are more than 50 symbologies used in the world today. Symbologies evolved over time for different applications, which is why there is more than one. The symbology most recognized is the U.P.C. (Universal Product Code) and its European counterpart EAN International (International Article Number). You've probably seen U.P.C. hundreds of times on grocery store and retail items. U.P.C./EAN is a numeric symbology. Look under the hood of your automobile, however, and you'll find Code 39, an alphanumeric symbology used for tracking, in this case, parts throughout the automotive industry. Fortunately, most industries — including health care — have narrowed the field by designating one or a few commonly accepted symbologies so that you don't have to choose from the complete roster.

In the United States, an organization known as AIM USA (Automatic Identification Manufacturers USA) tests, approves and maintains specifications for all bar code symbologies. As new symbologies are developed, they go before AIM's Bar Code Symbology Technical Committee for approval. In Europe, the European Committee for Standardisation (CEN) serves a similar function. The approved symbology specifications are used by manufacturers worldwide in the production of bar code printers and scanners. Thanks to this international foresight, you can be assured that bar code equipment is readily available that can print, read and process the symbology you use, as long as it is an approved symbology used appropriately.

Health Care Symbologies

The HIBCC originally recommended using the Code 39 symbology because of its data security and because the health care industry uses so much alphanumeric data. Other symbologies later accepted by the HIBCC are Code 128, Interleaved 2 of 5 (often used for shipping cartons), Code 49 and Code 16K. U.P.C./EAN also is an accepted health care symbology since many products manufactured for hospitals are sold in retail settings, as well. Today, many bar code manufacturers produce scanners which can read more than one symbology. This equipment is known as autodiscriminating, because it automatically identifies and selects between different symbologies. For example, materials management may receive products marked with a U.P.C. symbol or Code 39. With the autodiscriminating capability, all symbols can be read and decoded by the same scanner.

The creation of Codes 49 and 16K marked a change in health care symbologies. They offer the capability of encoding more information in less space. In addition to the usual patterns of bars and spaces used in traditional (also known as linear) bar codes, Codes 49 and 16K arrange bars and spaces in several stacked rows. These symbologies, referred to as stacked or two-dimensional (2-D) bar codes, have the advantage of storing more information than traditional linear symbologies.

Sample Codes

U.P.C.

Code 49

Code 39

PDF417

Recently, two new symbologies have been introduced and are being considered for health care applications. These symbologies, known as PDF417 (Portable Data File) and Data-Matrix, offer an even broader capability for information storage within a bar code. Traditional or linear bar codes act as a license plate. By scanning the code, the user quickly gains access to a set of information stored separately in a database. The new symbologies have the capacity to store a complete data set in the bar code. This new capability will be useful for applications requiring immediate and off-site access to large amounts of data. For example, bio-hazardous waste could be bar coded with PDF417 or DataMatrix so that the contents of the containers can be fully tracked at any location along its route to disposal. Not only would the bar code include identification information, as is included in a linear bar code, but it could also contain information on contents, special warnings, storage details, disposal instructions and critical dates.

How do you choose between the symbologies accepted in the health care industry? First, recognize the requirements of your application in two areas: whether you need an alphanumeric or numeric code and label size. Most health care applications require an alphanumeric code which narrows the options to four symbologies. The label size will also restrict applicable symbologies. For example, there is only room for a small bar code on a specimen or slide. Second, look at the symbology recommendations included in the application standards. Most bar code standards suggest one or two preferred symbologies. Third, take a look at the symbologies that appear on products coming into your organization from external sources. Finally, check with other health care institutions and see what symbologies they use for similar applications.

Summary

Symbologies are the language of bar code technology while standards are the grammar. To choose the appropriate standards and symbology for a particular application, you need to answer these questions:

- What information do we need to encode (what do our inputs and outputs need to be)?
- What is the recommended data structure for this application which best matches my information needs?
- What symbology(ies) is specified in the application standards for this use?

One final note: The HIBCC and the UCC are now collaborating in the development of additional health care standards. Be sure your technical staff checks the most current information about symbologies and standards as you prepare to develop and implement a bar code system in your institution.

If you are interested about organizations that are involved with symbology and standards development, more information is included in the Resources section beginning on page 123.

Bar Code Equipment: Decision Making Factors

Equipment decisions should be among the last made when implementing bar code technology. But planning a bar code system without understanding equipment fundamentals is like walking through a minefield. Take the example of a hospital that decided to purchase thousands of pre-printed bar code labels early in the planning process. Months later they purchased their scanning equipment only to discover that the equipment could not read their pre-printed labels. There was nothing wrong with the labels, nor with the scanning equipment. The hospital simply hadn't purchased the appropriate bar code labels for the reading equipment — a mistake that cost them. What the hospital should have done, was test the equipment by scanning sample labels to ensure equipment and label compatibility. By recognizing equipment options and requirements early in the process, you can make informed decisions that prevent costly mistakes.

In this chapter, we'll review basic bar code equipment needs — labels, printers and scanners. It is not designed to provide the technical depth required for making final purchasing decisions. Your technical team will need to do more research before selecting a specific product and manufacturer. However, the chapter will provide you with the overview decision makers need for system-wide equipment evaluation.

One caveat: Cost is inherently a criteria for purchasing any equipment, including bar code equipment. While it is not mentioned in each section of this chapter, it is certainly a key decision-making factor. However, it is important that the application — not budget — lead your equipment selection decision. Choosing the equipment that satisfies the requirements of your system needs to come first (i.e. printing small labels that will fit on a laboratory slide cannot be accomplished with a dot matrix printer). Once those decisions are made, there will be plenty of opportunity to select specific brands of equipment with a closer eye to budgetary constraints.

Labeling

How will tracked items be marked with a bar code? In some cases, products will arrive from the manufacturer already bar coded. Most hospital applications, however, require that you produce and apply labels as the information becomes available — to patients, files, x-rays, specimen tubes, IV bags, security badges, operating equipment, stock inventory shelves, medical records and more.

Making label decisions requires asking — and answering — a lot of pertinent questions:

- What textures and surfaces must the label adhere to: paper, metal, plastic, glass, wood, other?
- How many times a day will the label be scanned?
- How long does the label need to last? One day? Two days? Three weeks? Years?
- Will sequential bar code numbers be used or do you need to customize the information contained on each label?
- Will the label have to be applied to a curved or uneven surface?
- Does the label need to contain human readable information?
- Does the label need to contain graphics (i.e. a logo)?
- Will labels be exposed to liquids?
- Will the label be exposed to temperature extremes?
- Will the label be subject to abrasion?
- Should the label be removable or permanent?
- What glove material is used by people applying the labels?
- Do you need to write on the labels? With what?

- What type of scanners will be reading the bar code label: contact (the scanner touches the label) or non-contact (the scanner does not touch the label)?
- What kind of lead time is required between producing, applying and using the label?

By starting with the application, an effective, comprehensive range of questions can be evaluated before choosing the labeling method and/or equipment. Here's another hospital horror story exemplifying the importance of anticipating all labeling needs before making a purchasing decision: In one large hospital, the team involved with the system's development carefully defined their label information needs, but failed to attend to adhesive issues. After purchasing equipment, they proceeded to apply labels to all medical records used throughout the system. They finally began using their bar code system after months of labeling. As soon as records were pulled from shelves, labels began falling off. The team hadn't paid enough attention to their needs to anticipate and specify the permanent adhesive required for a medical records tracking system.

Consumer Power

When it comes to bar codes coming into health care settings from manufacturers or distributors, health care organizations have more power to demand quality than you may realize. One Illinois hospital had a problem with a supplier of hip joint replacement parts. The FDA requires tracking all implantable products used in replacement surgery. Typically, four or five sizes of a single part are taken into surgery so that the best size can be selected for the patient. The remaining parts are returned to inventory. In this case, hip joint replacement parts that had been bar coded by the supplier wouldn't scan. When the sales representative for the manufacturer was asked about the problem he said "Well, that's about as good as it's going to get." As a major consumer of health care products, you have the power to insist that manufacturers abide by your quality standards for bar codes. As you implement a bar code system, let suppliers know that you want bar codes at all levels of packaging (cartons, shelf packs and units of issue). Also let them know that you expect high-quality bar codes that conform to your standards and that read properly the first time they are scanned.

Once label needs have been identified, the remaining question is how will you acquire labels? Do you buy pre-printed from an external source or print labels internally? Most people assume that pre-printed labels are less costly than labels printed on-site. On the surface this may seem true, but it is important to evaluate your application fully before reaching this conclusion. Pre-printed labels can be an excellent choice for labels that can be purchased in large volumes, and which do not have to be patient-specific or printed using real time information. However, pre-printed labels may result in less savings for some applications and often add hidden costs in the form of inventory maintenance, productivity and waste. On-site printing may require a larger capital investment up front, but still provides a substantial financial payback as well as improving the quality and accuracy of patient-specific and time-critical information. On-site printing provides greater control over the content and quantity of labels you print. Additionally, it gives you absolute control over your labeling system. The point is this: Don't make any assumptions. Evaluate your label printing choices based on the requirements of each application and be sure to evaluate the long-term value of your options.

Bar Code Label Printers

Purchase decisions regarding bar code label printers are similar to those required when selecting a personal computer printer: The field of choices may be broad, but your printing needs lead you to the best value. Computer printers are selected based on the readability and lasting print quality of the output. For example, dot matrix printers create crude graphic images, so this type of printer would not be a good choice for a graphics department. And while laser printers create clearer letter forms, you may not need this high-quality typography for simple, internal applications. Similarly, different kinds of bar code label printers offer specific advantages and disadvantages depending upon their use. Knowing these factors will help you hone in on the best type of bar code label printer for your application.

There are three basic criteria for judging how well a bar code label printer suits your needs: label size, label quality and speed of throughput. The largest amount of information you need to encode in the bar code and the largest amount of human readable information you need drive the **label size**. This is also affected by symbology requirements, the number of characters of information you need to contain in the bar code. **Label quality** equates to the readability of the bar code. However, it is important to remember that this doesn't mean readability to the human eye, but how well and accurately the label can be read by a bar code scanner the first time and every time. **Speed of throughput** refers to the time it takes to format and print a label. It should be based upon whether you need a label delivered immediately (i.e. for a phlebotomist's draw list) or whether you have some lead time in generating labels (i.e. stock shelf labeling). High volume applications will often require speedier print capabilities, too.

Let's take a look at how bar code label printers measure up for label size, label quality and print speed. There are three basic categories for bar code label printers: dot matrix, laser and thermal.

Dot matrix printers use a series of pins that strike a ribbon against the label stock to form characters. Because they use multiple-pass ribbons, these printers must be monitored by an operator to ensure print quality. Dot matrix printers were not designed as bar code printers, so bar code quality is a consideration in choosing this equipment. The technology is not adequate for printing high-quality, very small bar codes such as those required for slides or patient wristbands. While dot matrix may be a good choice for some applications, such as forms, they are not the technology of choice for small labels or applications where speed and accuracy are required, such as on surgical joint replacement parts or in the emergency room. Dot matrix printers are also not the equipment of choice if printer noise is a limitation, such as in an intensive care unit.

Desktop laser printers are often used for printing bar code menus. Laser printing is similar in technology to that used in copy machines. A laser beam is scanned over a charged, photosensitive drum which takes on and transfers the image to a label. Desktop laser printers have the capacity to print high-quality bar codes in almost any size. Because they use 8½" x 11" sheets of paper, they are best suited for page-printed reports, such as bar coded pick lists, work orders and bar code menus. A bar code menu is a one-page sheet with multiple, bar coded information options. The user quickly scans items from the menu in order to capture the information. In health care, bar code menus are used frequently, such as when nurses record patient acuity, respiratory therapists track treatments and x-ray technicians develop x-ray reports. A bar code menu used for scheduling home care appointments, for example, could include bar coded options for the patient identification number, date, time, location, caregiver and treatment.

There are two types of **thermal** printers: direct thermal and thermal transfer. Both use a heat-induced system; the difference is that direct thermal printers use a specially treated paper for the process while thermal transfer printers use a treated ribbon with plain paper or synthetics. Thermal printers are designed expressly for on-demand printing, whether you need only one or multiple labels. This on-demand capability offers added security for ensuring the accuracy of patient-specific applications such as a pharmacist labeling a patient's prescription as soon as it is filled. Direct thermal and thermal transfer printers produce superior quality bar codes in all sizes — from bar codes small enough to fit on a slide to those big enough to fit on a chemical waste drum. Both also can print labels that accommodate a variety of environmental needs (i.e. temperature extremes, and contact with water, blood, alcohol and other solvents). Finally, you can find adhesives for almost any application using either direct thermal or thermal transfer printers. However, because adhesive requirements vary (i.e. adhesives for items going through an autoclave are not the same as adhesives used for frozen blood products), it is important to know the specifics of your application so that the right adhesive is recommended by your supplier.

Scanners

Deciding on a scanner should take place after or in conjunction with selecting a printer to ensure that the two pieces of equipment complement each other. Before discussing the different types of scanners, let's consider the key decision-making factors affecting scanning equipment purchases. First of all, you need to understand that a **bar code reader** and a **bar code scanner** are not interchangeable terms. A bar code scanner is the device that actually scans the bar code. A bar code reader is composed of a bar code scanner that is integrated with a decoder that links the scanner to the host computer.

Once again, you must determine which type of equipment will best meet your application needs by answering a series of questions:

• What is the distance between the label and the scanner?

- Is the label always in the same fixed position or will its position vary?
- What is the orientation of the label?
- What is the length of the bar code?
- Is the label durable enough to withstand frequent touching (contact) with the scanner?
- What is the light quality in the area where labels will be read? What is the ambient light quality?
- Can your label printer produce the bar code density needed in order to increase the read rate and accuracy?
- Do you need to record information in real time or batch time?

Once these questions are answered, you can define your scanner requirements. Scanners can be hand-held for flexibility and portability or mounted in a fixed position (i.e. the grocery store check-out scanner). Some scanners must touch the label as it's being scanned (contact scanners); others do not touch the label (non-contact scanners). In some cases, you may also want to choose between a fixed beam or a moving beam option. A fixed beam wand scanner conducts one scan per manual pass. With a moving beam laser scanner or CCD imaging scanner, multiple scans are conducted during one scan attempt in order to improve the equipment's ability to decode. Moving beam scanners are recommended for unattended applications in the data capture process, such as lab analyzers or a conveyor belt.

How Does a Scanner "See"?

All scanners actually read the reflectance of light off the surface of the bar code. In a bar code, the spaces reflect most of the light while the bars absorb most of the light. By measuring the difference between reflected and absorbed light, the scanner encodes information, which is decoded and reconverted into data once it is integrated into the host computer. That is why dark black bars and clear white spaces are best for ensuring bar code readability.

Now that you have a feel for the issues affecting scanner purchases, let's look at the three basic types of bar code scanners currently in the marketplace: **wands, lasers** and **charge-coupled devices**. Wands, also known as light pens, are handheld pencil-like instruments which are moved over the bar code. Wands are easy to use and easy to learn how to use with proper training. They are appropriate for low volume applications where accuracy is critical but speed of throughput is not. For example, wands are often used for scanning medical records. In some cases, wands are attached to small portable terminals (they look like calculators) so that information can be both scanned and key entered. Materials management often uses this combination in the process of taking inventory, restocking shelves and setting up exchange carts. A product number for each item on the exchange cart is scanned and the amount of inventory remaining is key entered. When the inventory is completed, the information is downloaded to the computer for immediate inventory reconciliation. A similar approach is used to capture information about patients, treatments and therapies provided in respiratory therapy departments.

A new generation of less costly laser and CCD scanners has dramatically reduced the cost difference between wands and moving beam scanners. Therefore, don't rule out these scanner options until you take a close look at the advantages and disadvantages of all three for the application under consideration.

Training Employees: It Makes a Difference

While wands are simple to use, the most frequent cause of wand errors stems from inadequate training. Here is a perfect example: A Nebraska hospital was not achieving the increased productivity they anticipated with a wand system. In fact, nurses were highly frustrated by the frequency with which they had to keep scanning labels to get a read. One day, an employee of a company that uses bar coding was visiting his mother in the hospital. Observing the nurse's frustration as she tried to scan several chargeable items, the visitor discovered the problem. The nurse failed to scan the bar code symbol from quiet zone to quiet zone (effective scanning depends upon scanning some of the white space at both ends of the bar code so that the scanner knows where the bar code starts and ends). Within minutes, the nurse mastered the correct technique and was able to scan labels accurately the first time. The next day, the visitor learned that the nurse had trained her colleagues. The nurse and the visitor had become heroes. This problem could easily have been avoided if proper training had been provided when the system was instituted.

Laser scanners offer the advantage of distance — they can read labels from the point of contact to a distance of fifteen or more feet from the scanner depending on the type of laser scanner being used. This makes them practical for applications throughout health care settings, such as in the warehouse or storerooms where items are stored on high shelves or in hard-to-reach places. Additionally, laser scanners can be used on curved or uneven surfaces, such as blood bags and patient wristband applications. Laser scanners are also useful when an item to be scanned is not being picked up, such as heavy books in the library, pallets and cartons at the receiving department and equipment maintenance. In fact, laser scanners provide an extra, quality control advantage when it comes to verifying biomedical equipment preventive maintenance. Scanning bar code labels placed inside the equipment assures that every step for preventive maintenance required by the JCAHO has been completed.

One important note: the type of lasers used in bar code scanners is extremely low wattage and presents no health or safety risk to the user. There is no relation between laser scanners and lasers used in laser surgery. In fact, research has proved that it is more dangerous to look directly into the sun than to have a beam from a laser bar code scanner strike you in the eye.

The third type of scanner is the **charge-coupled device** (CCD). Instead of registering the sequential differences in light, a CCD uses image technology to sense all the bars and spaces at one time. CCDs need to be touching or within inches of the bar code. CCDs also offer an added advantage for items that need to be scanned upright. In some cases, laboratories have fix mounted CCD scanners so that specimen tubes can be read vertically, which allows for scanning open tubes.

A Word about Hardware and Software

Hardware and software issues could make up a book by themselves. For the purposes of this publication, however, it is important to recognize that bar code equipment can be used in conjunction with most computer environments, from PCs to mainframes. Hardware for bar code technology can also be standalone or networked. In all likelihood, your existing hardware can be adapted for bar code use.

Technically, software is not bar code "equipment," but it cannot be ignored. Software integration links raw data obtained from the bar code readers to create the needed output. There are many existing software packages that can be applied in health care settings. The general rule of thumb for software is that if an "off-the-shelf" software program meets 80% of the need, it is unwise to start creating your own program from scratch. For many applications, however, health care institutions are likely to need customized software to integrate the application with other clinical, financial or management information. Many companies and consultants specialize in software integration. Be sure they have plenty of experience in bar code technology, clearly understand your applications and are able to discuss various hardware options with you. Many consultants who know bar coding don't understand the complexities of the health care environment, and many consultants who know health care have little to no experience with bar coding. Both are needed to devise an effective system, so ask a lot of questions before making any final decisions.

Summary

Selecting bar code equipment basically comes down to this: A bar code system cannot be effective if it doesn't work or people won't use it. Choosing bar code technology equipment hinges on one Golden Rule: Know Your Application. The application will drive your decision about whether to buy pre-printed labels or print labels on-site. The application will also help you determine what type of printing and scanning equipment meets your needs. Finally, don't forget that the best equipment alone will not assure a fully functioning system. For a system to work well, people need to understand its purpose and be well trained about how to use it.

Electronic Data Interchange: Taking Automatic Technologies to the Next Step

Electronic data interchange (EDI) is a communications technology that, when married to bar coding, creates a seamless, automated system for information management. Bar code technology automatically captures data for computer processing and manipulation. Electronic data interchange takes that information and automatically transmits it from the sender's computer to the receiver's computer and initiates a business process. EDI is most recognized for its purchasing uses — such as automatically transmitting purchase orders, delivery confirmations and invoices between suppliers/distributors and purchasers. In health care, however, EDI has also been used for electronic claims processing. (As of January 1, 1993, HCFA processes Medicare Part A and B payments in 14 days for electronic claims versus 27 days for claims submitted on paper.) In this chapter, we'll explore the tremendous potential of electronic data interchange for streamlining business, eliminating waste and saving costs.

What Is EDI?

Electronic data interchange allows trading partners to exchange business information electronically, which eliminates the need to manually re-enter data. There are three important concepts to understand about EDI. First, EDI's strength is its ability to electronically communicate between different computer systems.

EDI can be a particularly effective tool for linking applications within a health care setting, such as between hospital departments. However, its primary purpose is to speed information exchange between separate organizational entities. EDI is likely to play a significant role in the development of regional health delivery systems, because it can provide the link between hospitals, physician offices, outpatient and ambulatory care centers, managed care providers, insurance companies, long-term care settings and more.

Secondly, EDI is more than simply automating the flow of paper — it is a way of doing business. EDI does more than create an electronic document — it is an electronic process that takes place between two computers. EDI transactions do not require human intervention. The act of sending the transaction triggers a corresponding response. For example, the transmission of an electronic purchase order literally puts the delivery process in motion when it enters the receiving computer. In fact, some experts suggest that EDI should be considered an application-to-application exchange instead of a computer-to-computer exchange.

The third important concept inherent to EDI is that it assumes a standard format among all users. Universally accepted standards have been established for how the information is formatted, called ANSI X12. The standards do not control what is communicated, only the syntax, structure and content of transaction data. Options exist within the standard allowing trading partners to accommodate their specific needs. Like bar code symbologies, these standards guarantee that trading partners can "talk" to each other while maintaining the integrity and security of their own system.

EDI offers a broad range of benefits, many of which are consistent with desired reforms in the health care industry. EDI can have a positive effect on:

Timeliness. To say that EDI makes important information available faster is an understatement. In New York, the five-year-old Medicaid eligibility verification system validates patient eligibility immediately in much the same manner as a credit authorization occurs when using a charge card. The system has saved $10 million. In Massachusetts, a similar electronic Medicaid eligibility verification system has saved $9 million in the first year alone. By making the implementation of EDI for accounts payable a priority, the Veteran's Administration has been able to save more than $200,000 in discounts because invoices are now processed within the discount period.

Relationships. EDI builds more effective relationships with suppliers. As hospitals communicate daily product usage to suppliers, suppliers in turn can better anticipate inventory and supply requirements. One hospital that worked out relationships with suppliers used EDI to create a stockless hospital. The results included a reduction of 13 FTEs and the elimination of an off-site distribution center with an associated annual savings of $97,000. Additionally, the hospital realized better control of an additional 60% of the hospital's "unofficial" inventory, a reduction of 13,800 purchase orders annually, a reduction of 20,700 invoices annually and increased departmental capability (fill rates alone increased 4%). By applying the same concepts for improved relationships between players in regional health delivery systems, health care providers can improve communication and speed the process of quality care.

Accuracy. Like bar coding, EDI eliminates manual keying of information which can significantly reduce errors. Accurate information translates into accurate orders. When products are bar coded by suppliers, everyone is assured of accurate picking, delivery, receiving and issuing of the product. Electronic invoicing facilitates electronic reconciliation of orders to invoices. One organization using a manual system reported that of 200 invoices held for payment, 120 were held because of keystroke errors. Accurate communications between health care providers could significantly reduce the wasted time and costs associated with correcting errors.

Cost Savings. While the upfront investment in EDI can be substantial, the ongoing savings and efficiencies realized from the use of EDI can more than make up for the one-time expense. Eliminating paper processes, reducing errors and obtaining accurate information quickly allows hospitals to reduce or redeploy people and resources. Additionally, the automatic audit trail created by most EDI systems helps health care providers document their compliance with legislative and accreditation standards without additional cost.

How Much Can EDI Save?

- *It has been suggested that as much as 70% of printed computer output is re-keyed into another computer.*
- *About one quarter of the cost of executing a business transaction stems from data entry and re-keying.*
- *One company reduced the cost of cutting a purchase order from $50 to $5 by converting to EDI.*

The Marriage of Bar Coding and EDI

The marriage of bar code technology with EDI assures complete automation for many health care applications. Bar coding automates the *product flow*, so that it can be tracked, inventoried or validated. EDI automates the *process*, so that transactions based on product information can be made efficiently. By combining the two, organizations take full advantage of automation for quicker, more accurate data capture and data processing.

The chart on the next page shows the complementary characteristics of bar code technology and EDI for warehouse and inventory functions:

Bar Coding Characteristics	EDI Characteristics
• Accelerates incoming and outgoing product flow	• Accelerates incoming and outgoing information flow
• Expedites materials handling	• Eliminates paper handling
• Moves data faster within an organization	• Moves data faster between organizations
• Increases inventory control through reduced errors	• Increases inventory turnover through reduced order cycle times
• Improves warehousing and operational productivity	• Improves service and administration productivity
• Enhances Just-In-Time management	• Avoids "Just-In-Case" management
• Links the workforce to the computer	• Links customers and suppliers to the computer

SOURCE: Quad II.

Imagine how much more vital the speed and accuracy of data capture and processing are when the "product" is a patient. In one hospital, for example, nurses download information into the computer from scanned bar coded items automatically starts an EDI purchasing transaction. Products can literally be on the way to the hospital immediately after consumption. It is feasible that test results could be sent to physicians in their offices or other off-site locations for more immediate diagnosis and treatment around the clock. Ultimately, the time and effort saved through automatic data capture and processing gives health care exactly what the industry seeks: improved quality, increased productivity and better cost management.

History of EDI in Health Care

Like many technologies, electronic data interchange began in one industry and expanded to others. While EDI has been in existence since the late 1960s, cross-industry standards did not emerge until 1984. The earliest uses of EDI in health care were proprietary systems provided by manufacturers who were seeking a competitive advantage. Unfortunately, early proprietary systems did little more than shift the burden of data entry from the manufacturer to the hospital. Over time, more effective systems evolved that made a direct connection between the institution's inventory systems and the manufacturer's fulfillment operations.

In 1988, a task force established under the auspices of the Health Industry Distributors Association (HIDA) began developing a standard approach to EDI after recognizing that the proliferation of proprietary systems was burdensome and counterproductive. The work of the HIDA task force formed the foundation for broader-based efforts still underway by the HIBCC. A second organization, the Healthcare EDI Corporation (HEDIC), was formed in 1991 by 22 major hospital groups who are responsible for purchasing in 70% of all U.S. hospitals. The goal of the organization is to eliminate obstacles to the timely implementation of EDI in health care settings, including hospitals, HMOs, clinics, nursing homes and other health care facilities. By 1993, information networks devoted exclusively to health care information exchange were being created nationally.

How Does EDI Work?

While there are a number of technical layers to the EDI process, the general concept behind the technology is quite simple. (See Figure 6-1.) A company wanting to transact a business function with a supplier (e.g. placing a purchase order) extracts the needed data from its own application system. This data passes into translation software which converts the information into standard syntax. Communication equipment then sends the converted data via phone lines to the receiver's system. Once received, the data is interpreted by the receiver's translator into a file format which can be understood by the receiver's application system. Part of what makes EDI successful is the use of a standard syntax for communicating data, ANSI X12. Communications are translated into and out of X12 so that health care providers' com-

Figure 6-1: The EDI Process

1. Bar code labels scanned and data input to computer.

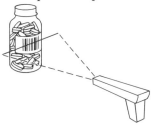

2. Information extracted from the sender's system.

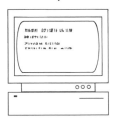

3. Information translated by translation software.

4. Information communicated from sender's system to VAN.

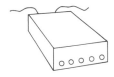

5. Information picked up by VAN.

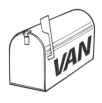

6. Information communicated from VAN to receiver's system.

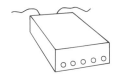

7. Information translated by translation software.

8. Information integrated into receiver's system.

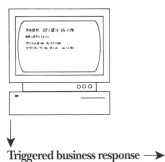

Triggered business response →

puters don't have to speak different languages to communicate with each trading partner.

Communications occur either by directly connecting one company's computer to the trading partner's computer or by using a communication intermediary called a value added network, or **VAN**. VANs function like an electronic postal system. You can log-on to a system 24 hours a day, 365 days a year and leave a **transaction set** (a transaction set contains information for one business transaction, such as an invoice or purchase order) in a mailbox on the VAN. Inter-VAN connections are also possible so that all trading partners don't have to be in the same VAN. VANs provide a buffer to prevent anyone accessing a system directly, which adds a layer of security.

It is important to emphasize that EDI occurs from application to application. Although sometimes referred to as EDI, E-mail and faxing are not forms of EDI since they do not trigger a computerized response. Additionally, if intermediary steps must be taken to manually key data at any point in the process, the advantages of EDI are greatly de-valued. That is why bar code technology dovetails so well with EDI.

Health Care Applications for EDI

Although health care applications in EDI began with purchasing and inventory functions, the need for reducing administrative costs in health care has shifted the emphasis to electronic claims processing. In October 1992, the Health Care Financing Administration ruled that all Medicare payments would be made either by transferring a check through regular mail channels or by direct deposit. In addition to limiting the modes of payment, HCFA requires providers who wish to receive electronic payments to submit 90% of their claims electronically and accept an electronic remittance advice. Clearly the government will no longer bear the cost of processing claims.

To avoid the new burdens created by this legislation, health care providers must be prepared to integrate their claims and remittance processes with EDI. As discussed earlier in this chapter, the states of Massachusetts and New York have already implemented electronic insurance eligibility verification and are experiencing dramatic savings. It is anticipated that other government agencies, such as the Food and Drug Administration, will soon follow suit and require information (i.e. outcomes measurements) to be submitted via EDI.

EDI will also play a critical role in linking health care providers and payers in regional systems of health care. (See Figure 6-2.) Computer-based Patient Records (See Chapter 8) are already in the formative stages and will allow patient information to be exchanged between hospitals, physician offices, outpatient centers, ambulatory care clinics, managed care providers, long-term care facilities and other health care agencies using EDI.

This will help streamline operations, eliminate duplication throughout a regional system, improve information access (leading to better clinical and management decision making) and reduce administrative costs.

Benefits for Health Care

Because of the unusual "product" in health care (the patient), EDI offers some unique benefits that mirror the industry's goals for measuring and achieving new standards for quality, improving productivity and managing health care costs better.

Quality
- Better clinical decision making deriving from immediate access to test/procedure results and other medical knowledge.
- Improved performance as a result of more efficient systems and increased staff morale.
- Greater patient satisfaction resulting from better clinical decision making and more time for personal care from doctors, nurses and technicians.
- Better compliance with JCAHO and other government reporting requirements.

Figure 6-2: Linking Health Care Delivery with EDI

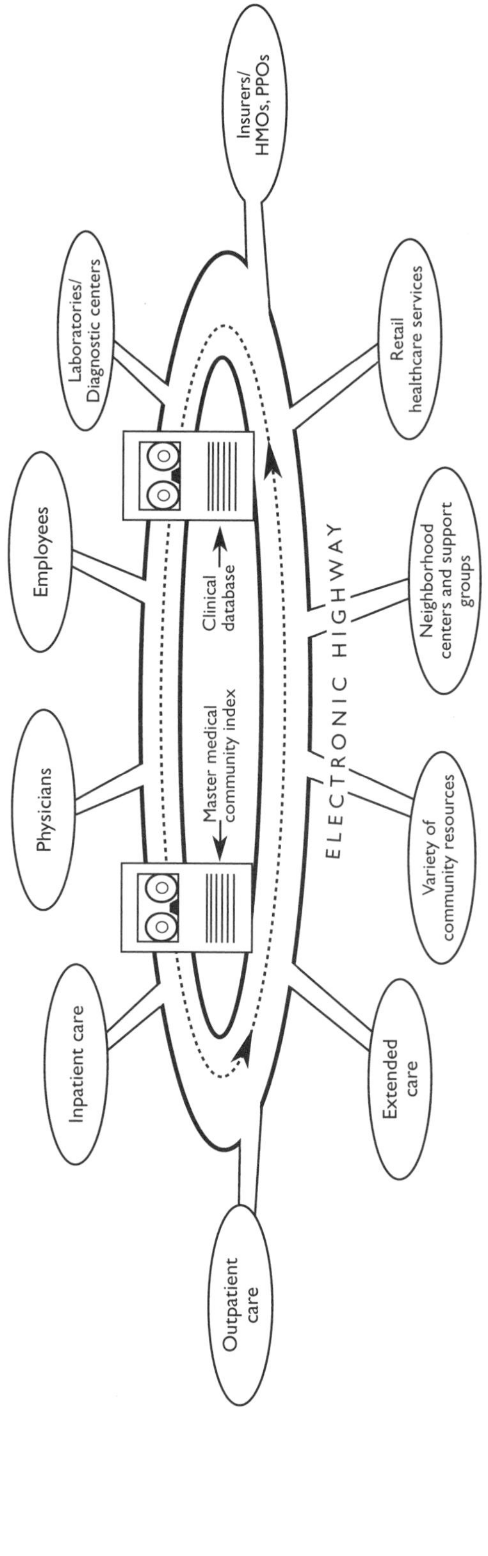

Laboratories/Diagnostic centers

Insurers/HMOs, PPOs

Employees

Physicians

Inpatient care

Outpatient care

Clinical database

Master medical community index

ELECTRONIC HIGHWAY

Retail healthcare services

Neighborhood centers and support groups

Variety of community resources

Extended care

Productivity

- Faster and more accurate delivery of medications and other supplies.
- More efficient scheduling of staff, resources and equipment.
- Quicker response time for procedures and test results.
- Less time and fewer FTEs spent on paperwork and claims processing.
- Better equipment and inventory management.
- More and better information available for clinical and management decision making.
- Better rapport between departments in a hospital and between all health care providers.

Cost Management

- Speedier reimbursement.
- Improved cash flow.
- Reduced number of days for accounts receivable.
- Significant reductions in re-submission of claims because of provider error.
- Cost savings from administrative streamlining, work reduction and improved inventory management.

Summary

Electronic data interchange automates business transactions between organizations. Using accepted standards, trading partners exchange information electronically for everything from purchase orders and invoices to verifying insurance eligibility and claims processing. Paperwork processes are virtually eliminated saving time, effort and cost. For health care, the marriage of bar code technology and EDI offers greater opportunity for achieving high quality care while maintaining cost efficiencies. Most importantly, the combination of bar code technology and EDI offers an ideal method for improving information exchange under health care reform in regional health care delivery systems.

Other Technologies: More Capabilities for Automatic Data Capture

Bar coding is just one of a spectrum of technologies that automate data capture. While bar coding is the most popular and widespread automatic data capture technology used in health care, other technologies offer certain features that may make them more appropriate for particular applications. Many of the automatic data capture technologies complement each other and become more effective when used in tandem. The purpose of this chapter is to provide a brief introduction to other automatic data capture technologies that have application in health care and their potential uses. The descriptions are not comprehensive nor technical — your staff will need to do more research about any one of these technologies. The descriptions are included simply to provide health care decision makers with basic knowledge about automatic data capture alternatives.

Radio Frequency Data Communications (RFDC)

RFDC is not itself an automatic data capture technology, but a useful complement to these systems. Using radio frequency, information that has been keyed or scanned into a portable device is relayed through a wireless system to the host computer. This allows workers to make real time decisions based on real time information. RFDC is most frequently found in manufacturing and distribution to assure Just-In-Time inventory management. Real time communications direct receiving, picking, put-away, shipping and cycle counting functions. RFDC has enjoyed success in health care for most of these same applications. RFDC is also an invaluable tool for improving clinical responsiveness. Current health care applications for RFDC include:

- In a number of hospitals, nurses capture patient information, such as vital signs and other assessment information, at bedside and relay it to the main nursing station in patient care units using RFDC.
- In a Toronto hospital, RFDC is used to manage exchange cart inventories and has resulted in a 50% reduction in inventory.
- The respiratory therapy unit of a 600-bed hospital in California uses RFDC in conjunction with hand-held units for data entry at the point of care, as well as decision support for analyzing and recommending appropriate therapies. The electronic system provides recommendations in five minutes that would have taken months to determine manually.

On-line, real time information is just one benefit of RFDC. Because these systems are wireless, they are ideal for situations where caregivers need mobility or operate at a distance from the host computer. RFDC also provides an inherent system for information verification or validation. The computer can relay a "wrong" message back to the caregiver before an error is made, such as in the process of drug administration. Finally, when RFDC is attached to an automatic data capture system like bar coding, it assures a completely paperless system, saving time and improving information accuracy and accessibility.

Radio Frequency Identification (RFID)

RFID uses radio frequency for identification purposes only. Tags with the capacity to send a radio frequency are attached to objects. When a tag is in range of what is known as a read station it transmits a signal to the receiver/transmitter. In some cases, a signal response can also be sent back to the computer. The technology is similar to the electronic article surveillance tags used in most retail clothing stores today to prevent shoplifting. (If you bring an item too close to the read station near the door, an alarm goes off.) Outside health care, RFID is primarily used for tracking items and for access and production control. For example, in some places toll booths are armed with RFID reading devices. As vehicles with RFID tags go through the toll booth, the system automatically deducts the fee for one toll from a pre-paid account, saving time and energy costs.

In health care, RFID is most widely known for two applications: RFID tags are placed on Alzheimer's patients to identify and track them in case they wander off, and newborn infants are tagged on the ankle to prevent any unauthorized person from removing a child from the nursery. Another form of RFID is **proximity cards**. Proximity cards use radio frequency to signal a reading station and provide access. They are a practical choice when the user's hands are busy. For example, doors between hospital units could automatically open for employees pushing gurneys that are tagged with proximity cards. The cards also protect security by preventing unauthorized personnel from entering restricted areas.

Memory Buttons

Memory button technology is relatively new and is referred to by a number of names: smart buttons, touch buttons, touch memory, data cells or data cans. Regardless of the name, the technology is the same — a small semiconductor chip contained in a stainless steel container. There are two types of memory buttons. The first uses a **simple chip** that is encoded with a serial number or other numeric code. Simple chips are used for quick identification and cross referencing. The second type of memory button uses a **smart chip** which can be electronically added to ("written to") by the user. The capacity of smart chips can be extensive. In health care, an entire patient record could be contained in one smart chip. Both kinds of chips can be reprogrammed for repeated use.

The portability and capabilities of memory buttons makes them appropriate for security uses, particularly lock control. For example, in a hospital, a memory button could be placed on a controlled substance cabinet and programmed so that only one user/device (known as a probe) can release the lock. Information about cabinet contents could also be stored in the memory button. A nurse must possess the correct, qualifying probe in order to open the cabinet. A bar code scanner on the other end of the probe allows the nurse to scan a bar code when the medication is removed. Using the probe, reduced inventory levels could also be registered into the memory button. Later, other personnel could read the memory button to obtain information for inventory management without jeopardizing security.

Another advantage of memory buttons is that they can be adjusted to download information directly from temperature, blood pressure, blood cell count and glucose gauges. This eliminates the need for any human intervention in documenting results at the same time that it validates the procedure. Memory buttons are being looked at closely to help health care providers document and satisfy Clinical Laboratory Improvement Amendments (CLIA) quality control regulations for bedside blood testing.

Voice Recognition Technology

Voice recognition technology is growing in appeal for hospitals because of capability and performance improvements. Voice recognition technology uses speech-activated computers to convert analog data (spoken words and sounds) into digital data (on and off bits). The digital data is compared to all the words the system knows, its **vocabulary**, to find a match. Recognition occurs when a match is made. Vocabularies for different systems can vary widely — from 50 to several thousand words. Usually the more words in the system's vocabulary the longer it takes for recognition.

Voice recognition technology is most appropriate in situations where the individual's hands and/or eyes are not free for data entry. For example, voice recognition technology is utilized in many emergency rooms to assure complete and accurate data capture for medical records without distracting doctors and nurses from providing emergency care. Anesthesiologists use voice recognition to record medical information during surgery which allows them to keep their hands and eyes free. Voice recognition is also a valuable tool in applications where the environment requires complete sterilization. The technology is expected to become more practical as manufacturers increase the capacity of systems to effectively process large vocabularies and to develop systems that are quicker and more accurate.

Pen-based Computing

Pen-based computing can be considered a subcategory of laptop and notebook computing. Instead of inputting information through the usual keyboard, information is input through a pen-like stylus by either tapping or writing on the screen. The portability of pen-based computing makes it useful for point-of-care applications. Pen-based computing is already proving its capabilities when used as an electronic clipboard for forms automation in hospitals. In a Kentucky hospital, nurses use pen-based computing to collect patient vital signs. Canadian doctors and dentists use pen-based computing to record medical assessments. Some pharmaceutical companies have given pen-based computers to their sales representatives so that they can capture the physician's signature at each sales call and release drug samples.

Theoretically, pen-based computing can also be programmed to automatically code input for ICD-9 (International Classification of Diseases codes) and CPT (Current Procedural Terminology codes) procedures. Once an order is written into the patient record, the computer automatically codes it for more accurate, automatic billing. Furthermore, in current applications pen-based computing has saved considerable time and money in transcriptions since the need for transcribing physician orders is eliminated. Research is being pursued to evaluate the appropriateness of pen-based computers for capturing electronic signatures for medical records (this is also contingent upon acceptance of electronic signatures).

Optical Mark Read

Optical mark read is a method for data capture that is most appropriately used with forms. You may not know the name of the technology, but you certainly are familiar with it. It's most commonly recognized as rows of circles representing options on a form where you fill in the appropriate circle to provide the correct response. Optical mark read is used extensively in the field of educational testing. At one time, only a number two pencil could be used to complete the forms. Now the technology accepts input from pens, pencils and markers. It also can be used in conjunction with bar codes to create a direct link between the information being captured and the patient. Optical mark read makes data entry for large amounts of information easier, faster and less costly than key-entry. Scanning data entry from forms can be up to 50 times faster with optical mark read.

In health care, the ability to enter large amounts of information into a computer quickly and accurately supports better clinical decision making. The technology appears to be most appropriate on forms offering an array of options, such as forms for lab test orders, treatment options or risk management reports. Current hospital applications for optical mark read include:

- labor and delivery notes for newborn babies by doctors and nurses,
- outpatient psychiatric intake records,
- health screening documentation,
- exchange cart items,
- physical plant maintenance,
- anesthesiology procedures in operating and recovery rooms,
- quality assurance and quality control in laboratories, and
- patient food menus.

Card Technologies

Identification cards already play an important role in health care delivery, and their use is expected to continue growing as these technologies improve. In health care, card technologies fall into two categories: those used for employee identification and those used for patient identification.

Employee cards are mostly used for time and attendance tracking and/or access/security control. There are two notable technologies used for employee identification:

Bar code cards use bar codes to identify employees. Access to areas in the facility or to certain items (i.e. narcotics) can also be controlled via bar coded employee badges.

Magnetic stripe cards encode data on a magnetic material that contains several tracks for storing information. (Magnetic stripe technology is commonly used on credit cards.) The cards are swiped through a reader and the identification information is compared to information in a computer. In addition to being used for security, magnetic stripe cards can function as pre-payment cards for services such as vending machines and cafeteria services.

"Patient cards" refers to card technologies used to store a certain amount of patient information. It has been suggested that the U.S. should adopt a national health care card program as part of new reforms, much like the program already legislated in Germany. While smart card technology has been selected in Germany, a data storage method for these cards in the U.S. has not been determined. Many health care providers are currently using embossed cards. In some cases, providers are implementing cards that contain a bar code or magnetic stripe. A few institutions have combined embossed cards with bar codes and/or magnetic stripes. However, a few more sophisticated technologies with greater information storage capacity are beginning to enter the health care arena. The term "smart cards" is often used as a catch-all phrase for any type of card technology. But, smart cards represent only one group in the spectrum of card technologies.

There are two recognized, more advanced technologies used for patient cards:

Smart cards, also known as integrated circuit (IC) cards, contain a small semiconductor chip with the capacity of a computer. Some European countries are using smart cards so that patients can carry a complete medical history with them wherever they go. Information can be easily changed and/or updated.

Optical memory cards use laser imaging technology to store information much like sounds and images are stored on laser discs. One of the key advantages to this technology is that it can incorporate graphics and visuals in the medical record (i.e. x-rays, CAT scans, warning symbols, etc.). Optical memory cards lead the pack when it comes to storage capacity; one optical memory card can hold up to 500 pages of information. A hospital in England has already implemented optical memory cards to track the progress of high-risk pregnancy patients throughout their terms.

Summary

While bar coding is the predominant automatic data capture technology in health care, it is not the only one available. Radio frequency data communications (RFDC), radio frequency identification (RFID), voice recognition, pen-based computing, optical mark read, memory buttons and card technologies all offer alternatives with distinct advantages and disadvantages. Many of these technologies complement each other and can be used in unison. Once again, if you know your application, it will lead you to the best technology.

If you would like to find out more about these and other automatic data capture technologies, please turn to the Resources section beginning on page 123.

Putting It All Together: Computer-based Patient Records

Throughout this book, the importance of knowing exactly what you want to accomplish has been repeatedly stressed. By determining the information needed, where to find it, how it is used and who will use it, health care executives can begin to make an educated decision about the best automatic data capture technology for the application. The strength of automatic technologies, however, comes into full focus when they are used in unison. In health care, Computer-based Patient Records (CPR) is an emerging application which best demonstrates the power of combining automatic technologies. CPR is a methodology for automating patient information already being used in some hospitals. Furthermore, CPR can't be ignored — there is good reason to believe that the use of electronic patient records may be mandated by law before the turn of the century. In this chapter, we'll review the current concepts and practices in CPR and demonstrate how automatic data capture technologies can be successfully integrated into this health care application.

What Is CPR?

The accepted definition for Computer-based Patient Records is "an electronic patient record that resides in a system specifically designed to support users by providing accessibility to complete and accurate data, alerts, reminders, clinical decision support systems, links to medical knowledge and other aids" (Institute of Medicine Study on Improving the Patient Record, April 1991). In plain language, CPR is more than just automating data capture and computerizing patient information — with CPR, patient records are computer-generated, computer-processed and computer-stored. For health care, bar coding and EDI make CPR both feasible and practical. Hospitals, managed care providers, physicians and insurance companies can derive and retain patient information from a single electronic patient record.

CPR is used for:

- patient identification,
- insurance eligibility and verification,
- retrieval of existing medical data,
- diagnostic and decision support,
- recording observations, orders and care-related information,
- records storage,
- automating billing and claims processing, and
- legal and accreditation compliance.

Reducing Liability with CPR

In many cases, hospitals lose liability lawsuits not because they did wrong, but because they can't prove that they did right. Medical records and other documentation may be incomplete or inadequate. Bar coding, EDI and electronic patient records offer an ideal solution to this costly problem.

Why Convert to CPR?

CPR has gained broad-based support in the government and among health care experts, providers and employers. Virtually everyone working in the health care industry struggles with the vast quantities of required paperwork. A quick look at the numbers explains why converting to CPR makes sense:

- 99% of patient records are currently kept on paper.
- At any given time, 30% of patient records are unavailable.
- Nurses spend approximately 30% of their time documenting direct care.
- An estimated 4 billion claims forms are processed each year.
- Accepted coding systems require the accurate use of vast numbers of codes:
  - 7,000 Current Procedural Terminology codes (CPT)
  - 15,000 International Classification of Disease codes (ICD-9)
  - 477 Diagnostic Related Groups (DRGs)
- The primary cause of lost malpractice suits for hospitals is the lack of adequate and/or available documentation.
- Hospitals have as many as one person for every five patients managing patient accounting functions.
- Federal and state billing regulations change frequently causing the inaccurate completion of claims. For example, in 1989, the State of Maryland and HCFA issued more than 200 billing and reimbursement procedure changes.
- Missing elements in patient histories and physicals can cost up to $6,000 per patient in lost reimbursement.

Projected Savings from CPR

Exactly how much can our nation save in health care expenditures a year using CPR? The projected answer is impressive:

- *$198.7 million saved in file clerk labor costs by automating hospital record keeping.*
- *$1.9 million saved through the reduction of inpatient hospital stays.*
- *$8.3 million saved through reductions in hospital/emergency room visits.*
- *$5 billion saved by electronically supplying diagnostic/education information to patients.*

Electronic patient records offer the specificity, speed and accuracy that is critical to improving health care quality, productivity and cost management. Timely and accurate quality measures help improve clinical and management decision making. Less paperwork allows employees to spend more time giving direct care. Speedier documentation saves time and effort. More accurate information assures charge capture, speeds claims processing and improves cash flow.

Paper Versus Electronic Patient Records

A comparison between a paper system and an electronic system of patient records sheds light on the advantages that can be derived from converting to CPR. Probably the greatest strength of a paper system is its familiarity — people are used to working with a paper record. Paper records also offer these strengths:

• easy to use and train,
• easy to customize,
• easy to add new data,
• flexibility for organizing data,
• accessibility at the point of care, and
• no down time.

However, advantages of paper records are offset by many disadvantages, particularly those reflecting inaccuracy, incompleteness and unavailability of information. The weaknesses of paper records include:

• data is missing, illegible and/or inaccurate,
• frequent misfiles and lost records limits information availability,
• bulkiness makes it hard to transport,
• requires a lot of staff time,
• expensive to use (forms printing and inventorying, form alterations and reprints, storage),
• data retrieval is slow, labor intensive and thus expensive,

- data aggregation is too expensive to offer outcomes measurements,
- fails to describe the patient experience adequately,
- lacks standardized definitions for terminology,
- format doesn't accommodate multiple problems over time,
- access is limited when patients are seen in more than one location and no link exists between inpatient and outpatient data,
- does not provide any links between providers,
- costs occur from warehousing records for years, and
- cannot interface with other clinical data.

Computer-based Patient Records respond to most of the shortcomings evidenced by paper patient record systems while maintaining many of the advantages. Advantages of CPR include:

- complete and accurate data available at all times,
- formation of a lifelong record for each patient,
- combines inpatient and outpatient data into one record,
- format elements developed based on the real needs of all health care-related organizations that may access the information over time,
- availability of decision analysis tools and risk assessments,
- links with medical knowledge databanks,
- links with other providers, insurance companies and employers as needed,
- user defined format for information — keeps it easy to use, and easy to train,
- ability to include outcomes measurements and other aggregate performance data,
- inclusion of video, graphics, expert systems, electronic mail and other technologies,
- accessible from all points of care,
- includes the patient experience, and
- reliable transmission of records over distances.

A major HMO tested computerized patient records with 250 of its physicians. The number of manually retrieved charts was reduced 59% with CPR, at an average cost of $5 to $10 per chart for the labor of retrieving, transporting and re-filing. Physicians included in the study believed that the quality of records rose 79%.

Costs for Converting to CPR

The cost of implementing a CPR system depends to a large extent upon the current technological environment within a health care setting and availability of funding resources. HCFA estimates that it will cost $39 billion to computerize the nation's clinical information. This includes investments by segments of the health care market as follows:

Health Care Segment	Unit Cost	Total Cost
Hospitals	$10,000 per bed	$12.14 billion
Physician offices	$20,000 per office	$ 7.22 billion
Clinical laboratories	$50,000 each	$ 300 million
HMOs	$90 per enrollee	$ 2.97 billion
Home health agencies	$2 per home visit	$ 582 million
Nursing homes	$ 1,000 per resident	$ 1.64 billion

To be conservative, HCFA doubled the figure to $80 billion, which still represents only 10% of current annual health expenditures. If the investment is spent over a period of eight years, every health care provider would have to spend between one percent and two percent of its operating costs per year on computer equipment — not an exorbitant amount when placed next to its potential savings and improvements.

Most experts in CPR development agree that costs for a systemwide conversion to CPR should be factored into reimbursement and payment schedules, supported by data users, divided among all who benefit, including health care consumers. You can expect regulation and legislation in the near future that addresses cost factors associated with CPR. However, it is important to understand that investing in CPR is not a short-term expense — the cost can only be justified over time.

Current Barriers to CPR

Exponential progress continues to be made in the development and implementation of CPR systems. Currently, different organizations are at different stages of integrating Computer-based Patient Records. Some hospitals have fully automated their medical records. Others are automating and integrating information within a given department, such as respiratory therapy. What is important is that any effort made to refine and automate systems using bar coding or other automatic data capture technologies supports an institution's movement toward CPR. By evaluating, streamlining and automating current records systems, health care organizations are taking the first step to prepare for CPR.

There are a few major stumbling blocks that must be overcome before CPR can achieve broad-based support. First, there are some technological limitations restricting the use of CPR. Computer systems still need to be developed with the power to manage the range and volume of information required. Second, standardized terminology must be developed so that information can be exchanged between organizations. This includes acceptance of standards for medical terminology, data naming and information formats, and a patient identification numbering system. Third, health care organizations exist at varying degrees of automation. Organizations will have to build up their technological capabilities to an equivalent level, requiring both the financial resources and the willingness to invest in CPR. Fourth, legislation and regulation needs to be developed in order to articulate rules for facility licensure; control, ownership and responsibility for patient records; computerization and storage of medical information; and protection of patient's confidentiality and rights. Finally, the cost of implementing and operating a CPR system is not yet factored into reimbursement schedules.

While these limitations make the current implementation of a CPR system prohibitive, there is much health care decision makers can do to prepare for the emergence of CPR. Automating and streamlining individual applications can help health care organizations put pieces in place that will eventually be linked into a CPR system. By adhering to existing health care technology standards and using automatic data capture technologies, you can create a solid foundation for future, electronic patient record systems.

Automatic Data Capture Technologies and CPR

Automating patient records is not a single application, but a myriad of applications woven together by flexible technology. That is why a complete system for CPR is likely to include different automatic data capture technologies. Figure 8-1 demonstrates the many ways bar coding and other automatic data capture technologies can work together to feed a CPR system in the case of a single patient.

In addition to these CPR applications, imagine the many other ways that bar coding and other automatic data capture technologies are working behind the scenes — for scheduling staff and resources, equipment maintenance and repair, purchasing and inventorying, management information, facility maintenance and hazardous waste management.

Figure 8-1: Sample of Automatic Data Capture Used for Computer-based Patient Records

Patient transported to hospital via ambulance	**Ambulance** Paramedics use **RFDC** to convey vitals to E.R.	
Patient enters E.R.	**Emergency** E.R. uses **voice recognition** to record activity.	
Patient receives bar coded wristband & is admitted	**Admissions** Admissions uses optical card provided by the spouse to obtain a medical history.	
Patient sent for tests	**Clinical Laboratory** Blood specimens drawn and **bar coded**. In lab, analyzers read the **bar code** to test specimens and report to E.R. **Radiology** X-rays taken and film jacket is **bar coded**.	
Patient sent to O.R.	**O.R.** Anesthesiologist records activity with **voice recognition**.	**Central Service** Supplies tracked & charges captured via **bar coding**.

(Continued on next page)

Figure 8-1: (continued)

Patient sent to I.C.U.	**Orders**	**Scheduling Tests**
	Drs. use **pen computing** to sign for orders. Nurses use **pen computing** to register patient acuity measures.	Tests & procedures scheduled via **bar coding**.
	Nursing	**Med Administration**
	Vital signs automatically downloaded to nursing station computer at regular intervals via **memory button.**	All meds are **bar code** scanned prior to administration.
	Pharmacy	**Reimbursement**
	Pharmacy dispenses meds using **bar coding**.	Charges captured via **bar code**.
Patient moved to a regular room	**Physician's Office**	**Pharmacy**
	Patient record transmitted back & forth to Dr's office via **EDI** for review and orders.	Pharmacy dispenses meds using **bar coding**.
	Nursing	**Med Administration**
	Nurses record patient acuity and convey data to the nursing station via **RFDC**.	All meds **bar code** scanned prior to administration.
Patient released	**Home Health Agency**	**Reimbursement**
	Dr's orders & patient record transmitted to home care agency via **EDI**.	System automatically classifies all procedures & treatments. Claims processed via **EDI**.

(This chart exemplifies the way bar coding and other automatic data capture technologies can be used to enhance electronic patient records. It is not all-inclusive and only reflects CPR for inpatient hospital care. The process would continue throughout the health delivery system, including the physician's office and the home health care agency.)

Summary

The movement toward Computer-based Patient Records is already underway. CPR uses automation to capture, generate, process and store patient information in place of paper records. With CPR, hospitals, physician offices, insurance companies, managed care organizations and other outpatient health care providers all input and retrieve information about a patient from the same computerized record. It is anticipated that large scale savings in time and costs can be realized through a fully implemented CPR system. However, there remain some developmental barriers to CPR, including determining how the cost for implementing CPR will be shared. Bar coding and other automatic data capture technologies play an important role in increasing the speed and accuracy with which information is input into a CPR system. Automating any patient-related application places hospitals on the road to CPR. Therefore, health care decision makers can move forward with bar code technology confidently, even before major steps are taken toward CPR.

Cost Justification: Dollars and Sense

Justifying the investment in a bar code system is more complicated for health care than most industries because so much of health care involves "intangible" factors. There are many hard costs that can help justify hospital applications, such as reducing paperwork, eliminating duplication and saving money. But in these days of quality assurance, control and measurement, the "soft" costs — improved quality and increased patient satisfaction — must be converted into hard costs. That means creating specific, tangible measures for what have traditionally been considered "intangible" factors. In this chapter, we'll look at the many ways investments in bar code applications can be justified with measures of quality, productivity and cost management.

Make It Measurable and Meaningful

A national survey in manufacturing companies identified the primary reasons why upper management rejected proposals for automatic data capture investments. The top two reasons were that proposals didn't meet investment criteria and that investment returns were not adequately quantified. Objective, quantifiable numbers are required to prove the value of any investment.

The key to successful cost justification for bar coding health care applications rests with your ability to create tangible measures for changes and results. Hard costs tend to be easy to measure — the number of dollars saved, the number of FTEs reduced, the number of square feet made available, etc. These kinds of tangible measures must be created for all costs, including those traditionally thought of as "soft" costs.

How do you create measures for something as abstract and subjective as "quality"? The answer is that quality means different things in different situations, and you need to obtain the input from the people using the application to determine exactly what defines a quality measure. For example, increased patient satisfaction is often considered a measure of quality care. Yet patient satisfaction differs for different individuals in the hospital. Patients may want:

- more individual time and attention from nurses,
- courteous, thorough and unobtrusive service from cleaning staff,
- tasty, eye-pleasing meals from foodservice,
- quick and gentle treatment from phlebotomists, and/or
- understandable communications and courtesy from doctors.

Each one of these requirements can be evaluated by different and specific measures:

Requirement	Measures
More individual time and attention from nurses	• Increase in % time nurses spend with patients • Increase in number of minutes nurses spend with each patient in an hour • % time nurse is in attendance for all uncomfortable or frightening tests/procedures • Decrease in the number of complaints by patients • % time nurses refer to patients by name
Courteous, thorough and unobtrusive service from cleaning staff	• % adherence to cleaning protocols* • Decrease in time it takes to clean the average room • Ratings of "Good" or above for housekeeping services from patients at the end of their stay

Requirement	Measures
Tasty, eye-pleasing meals from foodservice	• % adherence to quality control ratings for speed and temperature of meals served • % trays prepared according to hospital standards for foodservice* • Decrease in number of complaints about foodservice presentation and flavor • % average and above average ratings on daily patient survey
Quick and gentle treatment from phlebotomists	• % adherence to protocols that include making eye-contact and smiling at the patient when first greeting them* • Decrease in number of patient complaints • Decrease in misticks and specimen errors
Understandable communications and courtesy from doctors	• Increase in the number of times physicians greet patients with direct eye contact* • Increase in the number of times physicians ask patients how they feel on each visit* • Increase in the number of times patients who understand and can explain their illnesses/treatments to nurses prior to leaving the hospital* • Increase in the number of times physicians ask patients if they have any questions at the end of each visit*

*You and your staff will need to establish benchmarks for these measures.

The best way to create useful measures for less tangible benefits is to go through a thorough probing of those individuals who are currently involved with the application. For instance, if a nurse complains that the pharmacy is "no good" at responding to last-minute changes, ask the nurse what "no good" means. It could mean they are slow (requiring speed measures), inaccurate (requiring accuracy measures), unaware of the importance of requests (requiring measures of communications and under-standing), or demonstrate a lack of willingness to work in unison with the nurse (requiring identifying the source of the unwilling-ness and making behavioral changes before even addressing measures). Find out the real source or sources of the problem to find out what really needs to be measured. Then create a state-ment indicating how much you want to increase or decrease the result in order to define a specific measurement.

Other Justifications

- *The leading cause of failed blood transfu-sions is clerical error, accounting for the death of 200 patients annually.*
- *One in 433 data fields is entered incorrectly in blood banking.*

As your staff gets used to the process of identifying specifics, determining measures for speed, accuracy and reliability becomes relatively simple. These measures are critical for evaluating the comparative present and future value of every bar code applica-tion you implement. As a decision maker, however, you have to establish measures that respond to long-term strategic needs for your institution. Bar code technology, like all hospital-related issues, must be justified by how well it satisfies organizational needs. To accomplish this objective, measurements need to be articulated according to how they meet hospital goals. For exam-ple, the real value to the hospital of increasing speed, accuracy and reliability in claims processing is that it improves reimbursement and cash flow. Reducing the time nurses spend on paperwork can translate into improved patient satisfaction (stemming from more time spent with patients), increased capacity, reduced overtime for nurses and reduced labor costs. Bar coding health care applications needs to be justified both on the basis of tangible measures and on its ability to meet organizational needs.

Uncertainty Is the Real Enemy

No matter how certain you are of the new technology's benefits to your organization, support is needed throughout the institution. Uncertainty is the real enemy of any proposed technology change. As a change advocate, you should be able to respond to each of these uncertainties by offering supporting evidence for your cause:

- *Are business needs sufficiently defined to establish the actual necessity for change and/or value of projected change?*
- *Is the scope of the application clearly understood? Is project definition complete? Is internal support evident?*
- *Is the impact on (value to) the hospital, both good and bad, apparent?*
- *Is there any experience within the hospital with the new technology?*
- *How reliable is the proposed technology?*
- *What are the service needs for the new technology? What about availability of consulting, training, trouble shooting, system design and software preparation?*
- *Does the new technology offer repetitious benefits?*

> • *What does it cost to use the equipment?*
> *Is the equipment suited to its environment?*
> • *How easily will the technology be*
> *integrated into daily hospital practices?*

Health Care Justifications

Making your justification measurements tangible is a two-step process. First you need to look for every possible benefit of an application. Here is another example where involvement of those actually implementing the current system and who will use the new application can help. Their familiarity with the process and needs for improvement can help identify cost justifications. Encourage them to be comprehensive and creative in identifying the benefits of automating data capture for the application being considered.

Below is a list of common benefits for bar coding in health care, which can serve as a starting point for identifying the advantages of automating your applications. This list is not all-inclusive, but designed to serve as a springboard for your cost justification efforts.

Quality
• Better delivery of care
 – more time for caregivers to give care
 – error reductions for treatments/procedures
 – fewer misticks by phlebotomists
 – accurate dispensing of medications
 – improved staff satisfaction and morale
 – improved staff recruitment
 – reductions in staff turnover
• Quality assurance and quality control
 – availability of real time data where needed
 – increased accuracy in records and reporting
 – validation of patients for medication, test and procedure administration
 – improved risk management

Quality (continued)
- JCAHO compliance
  - more complete documentation
  - more accurate documentation
  - more accessible documentation
  - validation of patients for medication, test and procedure administration
  - validation of equipment and safety compliance
  - improved risk management

- Better clinical decision making
  - complete and accurate documentation
  - speedy availability of test results
  - more time spent with patients
  - accurate outcomes measurements
  - increased compliance with protocols
  - increased accessibility to medical knowledge

- Increased patient satisfaction
  - improved patient perceptions of care
  - increased patient referrals
  - responsiveness to patient needs

  - fewer care interruptions and errors
  - improved patient ratings
- Better equipment performance
  - more accurate equipment information
  - regular equipment maintenance
  - speediness of repairs
  - availability of parts as needed
  - improved supplier relationships
  - improved equipment safety

Productivity
- Increased speed and accuracy
  - timely availability of information (i.e. test results, medical history)
  - quicker data capture
  - improved through-put
  - improved response time
  - improved resource scheduling
  - improved resource utilization
  - more accurate documentation
  - more accurate test reporting
  - reduction in administrative errors
  - improved data consistency

Productivity (continued)
- reduction in waste and duplication

• Time savings
- increased capacity
- retention or reduction of current staff levels
- better use of personnel
- reduced overtime
- reduction in labor shortages
- improved through-put
- more time spent on direct patient care
- timely delivery of services
- reduced paperwork
- reduced documentation management
- streamlined operations
- better scheduling
- reduced time for waste and duplication
- ability to use Just-In-Time inventory methods
- increased inventory turnarounds
- reduced time spent on correcting errors

• Improved accountability
- streamlined operations
- more accurate documentation records
- improved JCAHO compliance documentation
- improved process verification/validation

- ability to trace supplies/materials/equipment back to suppliers
- improved staff morale

Cost Management
• Cost savings
- reduced/prevented lost charges
- reduced operational costs
- reduced staff turnover
- reduced equipment breakdowns through preventive maintenance
- reduced overtime and agency fees
- reduced labor costs
- reduced documentation costs (including cost of forms printing and inventorying)
- reduced malpractice costs (including malpractice insurance rates)
- reduced errors, including the cost to redo procedures
- reduced audit costs
- reduced storage/archival costs
- reduced duplication
- reduced waste

• Improved reimbursement
- more accurate claims submissions
- speedier claims submission
- accurate documentation to support challenges

Cost Management (continued)
- accessible information to support challenges
- increase in percentage of reimbursement
- increase in speed of reimbursement
- increase in amount of reimbursement

- Better financial management and stability
  - improved cash flow
  - improved, more accurate financial documentation
- increased speed and rate of reimbursement
- increased capacity
- ongoing cost savings
- improved inventory cost management
- improved relationships with suppliers
- more accurate billing
- timely availability of accurate operational cost information

Once you have identified all potential justifications, the next step is to attach measures to each. For example, when a nurse states that the application of a new technology will reduce time for administering drugs, ask the nurse how much time. Have the nurse provide an answer based on a typical employee's experience. Then use that information to develop a multiplier for forecasting departmental savings (i.e. number of nurses conducting the same task in the department each day). Later, these figures can be used to develop organization-wide justifications. If a person in plant operations claims an application will save money for repairs, ask how much money in the course of a year. Try to convert every justification you can think of into a number.

Other Justifications

- *Up to 55% of radiology reports cannot be accounted for at any one time.*
- *Some experts estimate up to 30% in lost charges due to data errors.*

Figures 9-1 and 9-2 provide examples of how to calculate justifications for the health care applications.

Figure 9-1
Time and Cost Savings from Lost-Record
Error-Reduction in Radiology

1. Total number of radiology files processed
   per shift _____

2. Percent lost files per shift
   (If you cannot formulate your own estimate,
   the national average is 30%.) _____

3. Total number of radiology files lost per shift
   (Line 1 x Line 2) _____

4. Estimated time for locating one lost file
   (in minutes) _____

5. Average employee cost per hour
   (To calculate, add the total salaries of all
   employees per shift [including fringe benefit
   and overhead factors] and divide by the number
   of employees.) _____

6. Cost for locating one radiology file
   (Line 4 x Line 5) _____

7. Cost for locating all lost files per shift
   (Line 3 x Line 6) _____

Figure 9-2
Time Saved in Documentation from
Automating Nursing Care in a Patient Care Unit

1. Number of hours per shift per nurse   8 hours

2. Percent of time spent on documentation per nurse*   30%
   (National average is 30%. Multiply Line 1 by .30)

3. Number of hours spent on documentation by nurse   2.4 hours
   (Line 1 x Line 2)

4. Percent time saved in documentation by bar coding†   15%
   (We'll use a 15% estimate. Multiply Line 1 x 15%)

5. Time saved in documentation by bar coding   1.2 hours
   (Line 1 x Line 4)

6. Number of hours saved in documentation by nurse   1.2 hours
   (Subtract Line 5 from Line 3)

7. Number of nurses per shift**   7 nurses

8. Total number of nursing hours saved per shift   8.4 hours
   (Multiply Line 6 x Line 7)***

* If possible, have nurses keep time sheets for two weeks and use real data for making this determination.
† Your MIS manager or consultant should be able to estimate time savings for the recommended system.
** If you collect real data, plug in the exact numbers for each nurse.
*** To calculate cost savings, multiply this number by the average cost per nurse per shift.

Comparative Measures

Health care is an industry that thrives on statistics, which can work to your advantage when creating cost justification measures. One type of useful measure is benchmarking, a comparison of your institution's performance in an area to other organizations. Resources from the American Hospital Association, the Health Care Financing Administration and other national organizations offer a wealth of information about hospital performance and costs (i.e. the number of FTEs in a particular department, the average daily salary of certain employees, percent of total budget expended on operations, etc.). You can compare your organization's performance to these statistics and then establish cost justification measures for improved performance by automating applications. You can also aggregate your own data and compare current to previous performance for a percent improvement.

A Process for Cost Justification

Creating cost justifications for most health care applications requires determining savings in time and cost. In this section, we'll look at a five-step process for justifying most bar code applications. The example used throughout this section is purchasing a routinely re-ordered item. The numbers used are for demonstration purposes only.

Step #1: Break down the process into its smallest parts. The more specific you are in isolating individual steps, the more you'll be able to streamline the process and derive more realistic measures of savings. Let's use purchasing as an example to demonstrate how this process works. A detailed breakdown of how a purchasing process could be represented* (from determining the need to paying the invoice) follows:

Task

1. Recognize the need
2. Identify the solution
3. Requisition and obtain approval
4. Contact purchasing
5. Shop for availability and price
6. Prepare purchase order
7. Place order
8. Track & expedite order
9. Receive & handle order
10. Verify receipt
11. Correct errors/problems
12. Verify invoice
13. Pay invoice

Step #2: Calculate the number of minutes it takes to complete each activity. Remember, different people may be doing different parts of the process, such as a nurse for Tasks 1 and 2, materials management staff for Task 3, purchasing staff for Task 7, receiving staff for Task 9 and accounting staff for Task 13. Be sure to identify each person separately. For simplicity sake, we'll limit the example to calculating time for nurses, purchasing and accounting:

★The breakdown in this example was developed with input from research conducted by W. W. Grainger.

99

Task	Time (in minutes)		
	Nurse	Purch.	Acct.
1. Recognize the need	2.00		
2. Identify the solution	5.00		
3. Requisition and obtain approval	5.00		
4. Contact purchasing	5.00		
5. Shop for availability and price		10.00	
6. Prepare purchase order		10.00	
7. Place order		5.00	
8. Track & expedite order		5.00	
9. Receive & handle order		5.00	
10. Verify receipt	5.00		
11. Correct errors/problems	2.00	5.00	
12. Verify invoice		5.00	7.00
13. Pay invoice			5.00
Total time	**24.00**	**45.00**	**12.00**

Step #3. Calculate the cost per minute for each type of staff-person you identified. This should include hourly pay, fringe benefits costs and an overhead factor. Add each column to determine the total number of minutes required for one purchase for each staffperson identified in the process.

	Nurse	Purch.	Acct.
(Hourly pay)	($ 30.00)	($15.00)	($15.00)
1. Pay per minute	.50	.25	.25
2. Fringe benefit factor (30%)	.15	.08	.08
3. Overhead factor (20%)	.10	.05	.05
Total costs per minute	**$0.75**	**$0.38**	**$0.38**

Step #4. Calculate the cost per purchase in staff time. Multiply each category by its cost per minute. Add these together to get the costs per purchase in staff time.

Task	Time (in minutes)			
	Nurse	Purch.	Acct.	Total
1. Recognize the need	2.00			
2. Identify the solution	5.00			
3. Requisition and obtain approval	5.00			
4. Contact purchasing	5.00			
5. Shop for availability and price		10.00		
6. Prepare purchase order		10.00		
7. Place order		5.00		
8. Track & expedite order		5.00		
9. Receive & handle order		5.00		
10. Verify receipt	5.00			
11. Correct errors/problems	2.00	5.00		
12. Verify invoice		5.00	7.00	
13. Pay invoice			5.00	
Total time	**24.00**	**45.00**	**12.00**	
Total costs per minute	x $.75	x $.38	x $.38	
Cost per purchase	**$25.00**	**$17.21**	**$ 4.56**	**$46.77**

Step #5. Project the anticipated time savings for each activity once a bar code system is installed in a second chart similar to the one in Step #2. Insert the same cost-per-minute figures calculated in Step #3 and multiply to obtain the new cost per purchase. Compare outcomes of Steps #4 and #5 to deduce projected savings.

Task	Time (in minutes)			
	Nurse	Purch.	Acct.	Total
1. Recognize the need	2.00			
2. Identify the solution	5.00			
3. Requisition and obtain approval	3.00			
4. Contact purchasing	1.00			
5. Shop for availability and price				
6. Prepare purchase order		3.00		
7. Place order		2.00		
8. Track & expedite order		2.00		
9. Receive & handle order		2.00		
10. Verify receipt	1.00	1.00		
11. Correct errors/problems	2.00	3.00		
12. Verify invoice		1.00	2.00	
13. Pay invoice			5.00	
Total time	**14.00**	**14.00**	**7.00**	
Total costs per minute	x $.75	x $.38	x $.38	
Cost per purchase	**$10.50**	**$ 5.32**	**$ 2.66**	**$18.48**

**Total projected savings achieved by
bar coding (60% savings)**

$46.77

−18.48

$28.29

This is the estimated savings for a single purchase by a single nurse on a single shift. Multiply it by all the items ordered by all nurses on all shifts and the savings become significantly more substantial. Then consider the additional savings for non-routine item ordering and orders from other staff (i.e. O.R. nurses, pharmacists) and the savings become enormous.

The last demand for cost justification is calculating the

anticipated return on investment. Three accounting techniques are typically used: payback, net present value and return-on-investment (ROI). **Payback** analysis is the easiest. It is used to determine when the money invested is earned back. Most health care bar code applications pay back in six to eighteen months. **Net present value** analysis is more sophisticated. It reflects the changing value of an investment based on time and the interest rate. **Return-on-investment** (ROI) analysis is the most objective of the three alternatives, but can overinflate the attractiveness of small investments. (Most computer spreadsheets can calculate return-on-investment and net present value.) Any one of the three techniques will give health care decision makers solid information for determining the ultimate economic gain of investing in a bar code application.

Charge Capture-A Perfect Example

No one in health care wants to admit that their institution is losing charges (a charge is the amount of cost for a product or service that can be reimbursed). But lost charges often have greater impact on institutions than most health care executives realize. Most health care experts believe that approximately 30% of reimbursable charges are never captured. Many providers argue that it is not worth the expense to create systems for tracking lost charges when they are only reimbursed at a 30% rate. Take a look at real numbers, however, and it quickly becomes obvious that capturing lost charges could significantly improve an organization's bottom line, particularly when institutions are operating at low margins.

Figure 9-3
Lost Charge Costs

	At 70% captured	At 90% captured	Gain
Net value	$20,000,000	$20,000,000	
Capture rate	x .70	x .90	
Total $ captured	$14,000,000	$18,000,00	$4,000,000
Dollars lost	$ 6,000,000	$ 2,000,000	
30% reimburse. rate	x .30	x .30	
Total $ lost in reimbursement	$ 1,800,000	$ 600,000	$1,200,000
Total gain			$5,200,000

For example, in Figure 9-3 a hospital pharmacy does $20 million worth of business a year. If only 70% of the charges are captured, it is losing $6 million. Besides losing this amount of money, the hospital loses the opportunity to be reimbursed against the larger amount ($20 million) and instead is reimbursed for only $14 million. With a 30% reimbursement rate, the additional loss in reimbursement is $1.8 million. But if the same hospital pharmacy increased its charge capture to 90%, it would reduce lost charges to $2 million (instead of $6 million) for a gain of $4 million. At the same reimbursement rate, it would lose $600,000 versus $1.8 million in reimbursements. That's an additional $5.2 million going into hospital coffers. Furthermore, the savings is annual, not a one-time experience.

Bar coding charge capture applications can go a long way toward solving this problem. An 800-bed hospital in the Midwest had been using a manual system for tracking narcotics charges. They invested $78,000 in a system that uses bar coding for data capture, including charge capture. Not only did they achieve payback in a matter of weeks, but annual charge capture for narcotics increased to $3 million and they brought in a net revenue of $72,000 in one year. Better charge capture not only increases the bottom line, it also provides decision makers with the real information they need to negotiate contracts with employers and managed care providers and to make effective management decisions.

A Final Word

Regardless of the method of analysis you choose, the objective for cost justification is always the same: to take the emotion out of decision making when considering an investment in bar coding. Objective measures are easier to track and compare without worrying about the stake that individuals may or may not have in the success of an application.

When it comes to cost justification, however, there is one last valuable word of advice — as important as it is to create objective measures, it is also important to know when to stop trying to justify an application and just do it. Finding the one "right" justification can go on forever, and a bar code system will only work if it is put into effect. Follow the procedures outlined in this chapter to make objective calculations for the value of investing in bar coding applications, but set a limit. Use your judgment as a decision maker and leader to know when to draw the line on calculations and when it is time for action.

Other Justifications

- *For some health care applications, a 99% accuracy rate may not be accurate enough. For example, in laboratories, a 1% error rate for an average of 1.8 million lab tests processed a year equates to 18,000 errors a year.*
- *The error rate for human keystroke operators is approximately 1 in 300. Bar code technology errors occur less often than 1 in 3 million characters.*

Summary

Like all business decisions, the cost of investing in bar code technology needs to be evaluated. The key for bar coding is to create tangible, objective measures for every proposed benefit of the system — especially those that justify "soft" costs such as quality. Objective measures must also be made meaningful by showing how the benefits align with organizational needs and priorities. Payback, net present value or return-on-investment analysis should be used for the final economic justification. Most importantly, be sure to know when to stop the process of calculating benefits and when to start experiencing benefits by putting the system in place.

Making It Work: Preparing for Successful Health Care Applications

Understanding the vast and specific potential of bar code technology is only half the battle in moving forward with automatic data capture. Equally important is the process health care organizations use for evaluating needs, articulating systems, selecting equipment and integrating the technology into daily operations. In this chapter, we'll review a preferred implementation process for bar coding health care applications and identify common barriers to success.

Rules of the Road

For health care institutions, as with most organizations, there are two immutable rules for effectively automating data capture with bar code technology:

Rule #1 — Obtain top management commitment for bringing the technology into the organization. Remember that bar code technology tracks information. In a health care setting, information travels from department to department following the patient's pathway, requiring a broader outlook. An organizational perspective for technology selection is also more cost effective and less time consuming in the long run, because implications for expanding technology use can be planned into the system from its inception. The involvement of the institution's chief executive, financial and information officers ensures that all present and future exigencies are considered before financial commitments are made. Top level commitment also signals the importance and seriousness of this change to all staff.

In some cases, an operational manager recognizes the technology's potential when upper management lacks the vision. There are examples of hospitals that have met with a degree of success despite a laissez-faire attitude from top management. This is particularly true in cases of self-contained applications limited to a department. However, while these practices show positive benefits and results, they do not take advantage of bar coding's broader potential for greater efficiency and cost savings. The most successful applications (those producing the biggest savings in dollars, productivity and quality) in all industries are applications which have received a clear commitment from top management.

Rule #2 — Form a team to manage the process of change.
Integrating bar code technology into health care applications requires more than just automating current processes. The organization's evaluation must be grounded upon careful investigation and revision of current systems. After all, bar code technology is just a tool, and like all technologies it depends upon the quality of the information input. The goal is to streamline processes. If extraneous, incomplete, or erroneous information is entered into a bar coded system, it is impossible to achieve improved output and/or greater efficiencies.

The best individuals to evaluate a system are the people who manage the information now and will use the technology in the future. Because health care information crosses departmental boundaries, the project team should include directors from each of the major departments (nursing, medical staff, medical records, pharmacy, management information systems, materials management, radiology, laboratory, plant management). Upper management needs to be involved in assuring the program's consistency with long-range and short-range goals. The role of MIS is to serve as technical experts offering support in identifying the best technology(ies) once system users have clearly identified needs. Additionally, technical professionals will have to participate in order to structure the technical parameters around existing health care management information systems.

It is critical for the project team to have a leader. This person champions the cause of automating data capture systems with bar code technology throughout the organization, keeps the project team on schedule, holds accountability for progress, and serves as a long-term advisor for technology improvements. Someone must be empowered with the responsibility and authority of bar code coordinator in order for the process to function effectively. Hospitals with chief information officers usually make this person the bar code coordinator.

The bar code coordinator and upper management should define the purpose of the process, set goals and create a preliminary timeline before the project team meets. Then, a Bar Code Committee should be established and be charged with responsibility for setting priorities, determining accountabilities, managing the project, and providing visibility for bar coding applications throughout the institution.

At the first meeting of the Bar Code Committee, the bar code coordinator must set the tenor of the project by presenting:

- management goals and requirements,
- team members and their responsibilities,
- background on the project's inception and current state of technology use,
- parameters and expectations for the project (i.e. timeframe, budget),
- resource availability,
- task assignments for each participant, and
- expected information for the next meeting.

Once the Committee has been formulated, all members need to be educated to bring everyone up to a common level of knowledge about the technology and its benefits. Then the team must undertake a disciplined process to assess institutional and departmental needs, identify equipment and software preferences, plan a long-range strategy, create a budget and timetable for implementation, develop an educational training program and execute the implementation plan.

What Doesn't Work

Studying the characteristics of failed programs can be as valuable as studying successful programs. Failed programs can be characterized by a number of common traits:

- There is no clear commitment from upper management and/or support for the team.
- A "team spirit" is never formulated. In some cases, this takes the form of one department (most commonly MIS) dominating the program and excluding the other team members from significant participation. In other cases, participants only stand up for their own needs without trying to understand or support their counterparts. If project team members can't get along, the program won't progress.
- The organization fails to adapt to the new technology, because it lacks a clear, consistent commitment to the program.
- Team members fear taking action because of internal politics or their discomfort with the technology and investment. The Bar Code Committee and its chair must be imbued with real power to make bottom-line decisions for the organization.
- A corollary to the above is lack of buy-in from all levels of the organization. Any one level — upper management, middle management, operational management or staff — can undermine the entire program if they are not convinced of the program's benefits to them.
- Too much focus is placed on the technology and not enough on the reasons for using the technology (system benefits).
- Staff is unwilling to work with other departments. For example, developing a successful drug administration program requires that pharmacy and nursing work together.
- Training is not perpetuated. Early enthusiasm can bring impressive results, but the real test of the system is in the long haul. Programs that do not take refresher training into account tend to loose momentum.

Success is predicated upon six key factors. Hospital staff must:

- feel they own the project,
- view the programs' goals as achievable and support the goals,
- make the system part of daily operations,
- take initiative,
- change with changing conditions, and
- use available resources.

Needs Assessment

To assure that the new systems will provide the efficiencies needed, thorough institutional and departmental assessments must be conducted to establish effective long-range strategies. In addition to completing a thorough analysis, the institutional assessment serves as a valuable awareness builder. This is your opportunity to look for organization-wide opportunities and potential efficiencies. The institutional assessment should include:

- evaluation of possible applications, efficiencies and benefits in all areas,
- determination of computer usage, availability and interfaces for applications under consideration,
- calculation of the impact of bar coding, both financially and non-financially (see Chapter 9 for more information about cost justification), and
- identification of interested individuals on all levels who are willing to participate in the development, testing and refinement of bar code applications and help stimulate the interest and support of their peers.

The departmental assessment demands the most fastidious analysis. To evaluate needs on a departmental level, team members must be able to look beyond the existing system and seek the true, underlying purpose(s) for each application. Departmental staff should be pulled into the team at this stage since they are most familiar with the tasks at hand.

Defining "purpose" is rarely as obvious at it first appears. For example, most people might conclude that the purpose of improved systems in a clinical laboratory is more efficient testing. But a clinical laboratory does not exist merely to conduct tests — its underlying purpose is to provide important information. A more accurate reflection of a clinical laboratory application's purpose might be to speed information reporting and access, improve clinical decision making or increase capacity.

Once departments have defined the purpose, the next step is to determine how it can be accomplished. To do this, the team needs to take the entire application and break it into its smallest components. Develop a flow chart modeling all the alternative choices throughout the process. Document who gets involved, when, and how information is communicated. Flowcharts make the process easier to see and easier to assess. The flowchart on page 113 is an example of how one hospital processed drug administration on a patient unit.

The next task is probably the most difficult — evaluating how the process could be accomplished in other ways. Most automatic data capture professionals will tell you that it is easier to create a new system than to change an existing one. Experience shows that automating a bad system may speed the process, but ultimately will not achieve the benefits health care organizations need. This is your organization's opportunity to redefine the system.

One helpful indicator of possible change is the path of paper. Is there paperwork (or steps) that can be eliminated? Is there paperwork (or steps) that can be streamlined? Does part of the application take too long? Is information being reconstructed when it enters another department? Be sure to ask the people executing the system for their input — they'll know what does and doesn't work the best. Then take some time to use research and creative brainstorming techniques to envision different systems. This should include thinking about opportunities that a new system could generate. Can you construct a new system that generates reports, validates activities or offers an evaluation not presently available? Finally, talk to other health care organizations using the technology to see how they have structured their process.

Figure 10-1: Flowchart Illustrating Drug Administration Process on a Patient Care Unit

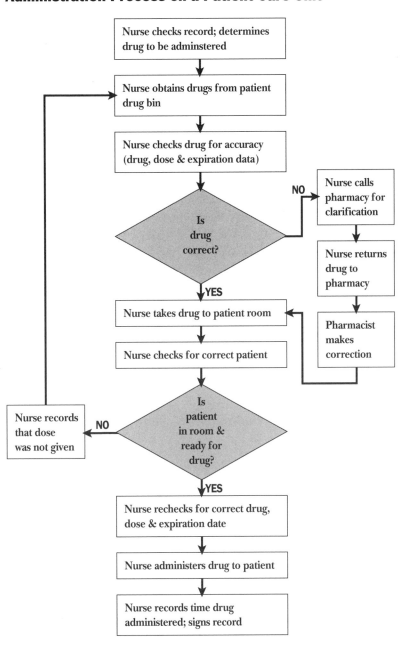

SOURCE: Yvone Abdoo, PhD., RN, University of Michigan School of Nursing.

Departments assessing their bar code needs should ask themselves questions for each application, such as:

- How will the information be used? By whom?
- What does the information need to look like in the end?
- Where does the beginning information come from?
- Where does the information need to be collected?
- How quickly does the information need to be made available?
- What other systems does this application need to tie in to?
- Who else in the organization could use (benefit from) this information?
- Does the information cross into other departments?
- Are the same terms being used within the department? Between departments?
- Can we alleviate the need for other departments to re-key patient information we are inputting to the system (i.e. patient name, patient identification)?
- What external documentation is needed (i.e. for the Health Care Financing Administration, third party payers, Joint Commission on the Accreditation of Healthcare Organizations, Occupational Safety and Health Administration, Environmental Protection Agency, Food & Drug Administration, etc.)?

Identifying Technical Requirements

Choosing the appropriate hardware and software for your bar code application needs is usually a complex, technical decision-making process which may require outside expertise. However, there are some important guidelines that will prepare the team and technical staff for choosing equipment and possibly a consultant.

First of all, remember the Golden Rule: It is critical to let the application drive the equipment choice. All too frequently organizations rush out and purchase hardware they think they need. This can be particularly counterproductive in a health care organization where the nuances of each application can vary dramatically. One department's hardware needs may be significantly different (which does not necessarily mean more expensive) than another because of subtleties of use. The key is to evaluate your need first and let the application suggest the best choice of equipment (see Chapter 5 for more information about bar code equipment and hardware considerations). The bar code coordinator can facilitate coordination and connectivity between systems and applications.

Using a Technical Consultant

Because of the range of alternatives and technical complexities associated with bar coding, technical consultants can be helpful in developing a health care program. Consultants offer experience, technical knowledge, and supplier relationships that can reduce risks and give you a better chance of implementing the right program the first time.

Here are some guidelines for working with a technical consultant:
- *Find someone who is experienced with your health care application.*
- *Consider a consultant who is familiar with your existing and proposed equipment.*
- *Seek a consultant who has proven contacts with bar code equipment suppliers.*
- *Involve the consultant as early in the process as possible.*
- *Use the consultant in an advisory capacity. Don't expect to dump the whole project in his/her lap. Remember, it is important for staff to evaluate and create the underlying system. Let the consultant advise you on technical matters.*

> • *Maintain a collaborative and managerial relationship between the chairperson and the consultant.*
>
> • *Don't base selection of a consultant strictly on price. Experience, familiarity, contacts and good chemistry will save you money in the long run.*

Secondly, be sure any outside support you receive comes from individuals who have used the equipment. Many health care organizations want to turn to their suppliers of hospital information systems and clinical information systems for support in identifying and purchasing bar code equipment. Many of these groups can supply the equipment but have little experience using it and, therefore, may not recognize expansion opportunities. Whether you are working with a familiar vendor or a new consultant, be sure the individual is educated about the specific equipment and application you are evaluating.

Departmental analysis provides the basis for determining your software requirements. For each application considered, you need to know:

General system parameters. What are the limitations and constraints of your system? Who will use the technology? Are there any outside vendors who will interface with your system? What constitutes adequate response time?

Existing computer capabilities. How much memory do you have available for a proposed application? Is it enough? Do you need more? Can your computer be upgraded? How much would additional capacity cost? Is your system networked? Does it have open access or is security protected? What contingency is available if the system goes down? What contingency is available if the bar code printer or scanner goes down? (Note: Bar code systems can interface effectively with personal, mini, and mainframe computers.)

Requirements for management reports. What information will result from tracking, inventorying or validating this information? Who needs to see the information? For what purpose(s)? The objective here is not necessarily to collect more data and create more reports (there is such a thing as too much information), but to establish an effective system for documenting and reporting needed information.

Planning a Long-range Strategy

A long-range strategy must balance the organization's long-term information and technology needs with the varying needs of each departments. Having collected and shared the departmental assessments, the Committee must now decide what applications to fund and in what order. In some cases, applications may require that two or more departments get up and running at the same time (i.e. admissions and pharmacy).

Each department should offer a justification for its applications using the measures explained in Chapter 9. Some of the applications will suggest a natural order. For example, admissions needs to produce a bar coded wristband before anyone can validate medications being administered. The Committee should be sure that the first selections are small, definable applications you know will result in success. These success stories can be leveraged for additional buy-in by staff.

For each selected application, the Committee needs to establish a budget and timeframe. In developing budgets, it usually is beneficial to be conservative when predicting savings. The timeline must include pilot project training and implementation, a completion audit that assesses hardware, software, output, usage, problems, reactions, etc., and program/application expansion.

Figure 10-2
Sample Timeline

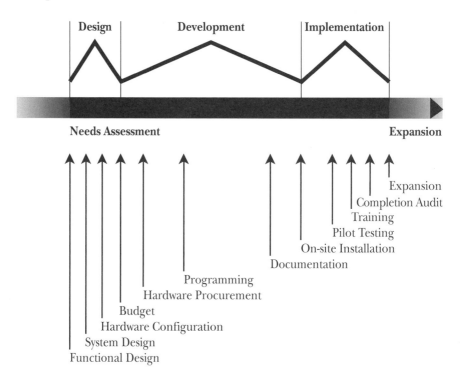

Developing an Educational/Training Program

Like most changes, the move to bar code technology is often met with fear and resistance. People are concerned about how changes will affect their jobs — how much more work it may require, the technical complexity of the equipment, and the possibility of having their work more closely documented and reviewed by management. The best way to overcome this resistance is to keep all staff informed about the decisions being made from the very beginning of the project. Knowing the purpose and activity surrounding bar coding applications gives staff an opportunity to understand the need and participate in the implementation process as early as possible.

From the system's inception, the project team should plan ongoing communications to build support throughout the institution. Department directors should involve staff in defining the procedures and desired outcomes for departmental assessments. The goal is to let the people using a technology decide how it can best be used. After all, who knows better about the system and information needs than the people collecting and reviewing the information? Any individual demonstrating interest should be encouraged to participate more. Staff should be informed of progress regularly through internal newsletters or memos.

Training Works

Whether concerns are large or small, real or perceived, every successful bar code system uses training to overcome staff misunderstandings and fears. By addressing real and perceived staff objections up front, you can avoid some costly problems later. For example, in a large Midwestern hospital, one nurse was afraid to scan a bar coded menu for patient acuity weeks after receiving training. She simply refused to use the technology. Finally, her manager and the bar code coordinator sat her down and got her to admit to the problem: She thought if she did something wrong when she scanned a bar code the entire system would crash. Thorough training could have addressed and allayed this unrealistic fear preventing the many weeks of lost time.

Training can significantly improve the effective utilization of a bar code system. The Bar Code Committee should be sure to develop an educational/training program before installing equipment. For each application, assemble any staff that will be involved with a system. Explain the purpose of the new technology and system. Emphasize benefits to the institution; the same benefits you used to justify the expenditure. Also emphasize the benefits to the user, such as easing stress, offering quicker information, providing more flexibility, etc. For example, bar coding hazardous waste can alleviate pressures on staff by eliminating their responsibility for managing paperwork and small, but important, details.

In the course of education and training, be sure to set staff's expectations for change by defining the transitional period and the time it takes for an individual to master the technology. Extended transition periods are not recommended because they tend to increase fears and lead to duplication and waste. A physical demonstration of the equipment, however, is recommended, because the opportunity to touch and use the equipment often helps alleviate fears. Consider developing a video demonstration how the bar code application works and its benefits. During and after the training period, make the bar code equipment available for staff to play with before making the conversion. Finally, give staff the name of a resource person or persons who can answer any questions on a daily basis.

After completing all this preparation, the final challenge is implementation. Typically the implementation process includes educating management, staff demonstrations, installation of hardware, test applications, training workers, converting to the new applications, recording and quantifying actual benefits, obtaining feedback and enhancing applications.

Training and education cannot be a one-shot deal. Ongoing feedback and refresher training are the cornerstones to successful long-term programs. After about three to four weeks, the Bar Code Committee should reassemble staff to obtain their feedback. Perhaps the equipment is not well located. Maybe steps have been left out. Someone may have an improvement or even an unexpected extension for the technology's use. User feedback is invaluable in assuring optimum efficiency of the bar code system. This also provides another opportunity to overcome any remaining resistance.

Refresher training is another significant factor in the success of automatic data capture. Laxity in something as simple as learning the proper way to use a wand can make measurable differences in data integrity and results. To avoid complacency, staff should participate in periodic refresher training, especially when new steps are added or applications are expanded. This also provides a structure for introducing new applications. Education and training should also include development of an introductory program for new and/or transferred employees and for temporary and contract employees.

Summary

Effective integration of bar code technology in health care settings requires top management support and a coordinated team effort. Representatives of every department should be involved in assessing current systems and recommending improvements and opportunities. A Bar Code Committee ushers the process through the organization and decides which applications to support, in what order, in what timeframe, and with what budget. The Committee is also responsible for justifying the project to upper management, technical professionals, department directors and staff. Education and training are integral components to implementation, as are evaluation and feedback. Once the program is in place, the bar code coordinator continues to manage system changes and improvements.

The principles described in this chapter apply to implementing any automatic data capture technology and electronic data interchange. By following these steps and The Golden Rule of Bar Coding (Know Your Application), you can find countless ways for bar code technology to help you improve health care delivery in your institution during the coming years of health care reform.

Resources

Organizations

AIM USA (Automatic Identification Manufacturers USA)
634 Alpha Drive
Pittsburgh, Pennsylvania 15238-2802

ASTM (American Society for Testing and Materials)
1916 Race Street
Philadelphia, Pennsylvania 19103

American Hospital Association (AHA)
840 N. Lake Shore Drive
Chicago, Illinois 60611

American National Standards Institute (ANSI)
1430 Broadway
New York, New York 10018

Commission for European Normalization (CEN)
36 Rue de Stassart
B-1050 Bruxelles - Belgium

Computer-Based Patient Record Institute, Inc. (CPRI)
c/o American Health Information Management Association
919 N. Michigan Avenue, Suite 1400
Chicago, Illinois 60611

**European Health Industry Business
Communications Council (EHIBCC)**
Boulevard Louis Schmidt 87, Box 3
1040 Brussels - Belgium

Healthcare EDI Corporation (HEDIC)
1405 N. Pierce, Suite 100
Little Rock, Arkansas 72207

Health Industry Business Communications Council (HIBCC)
5110 N. 40th Street, Suite 250
Phoenix, Arizona 85018

Health Industry Distributors Association (HIDA)
225 Remekers Lane, Suite 650
Alexandria, Virginia 22314

Health Industry Manufacturers Association (HIMA)
1030 15th Street N.W.
Washington, DC 20005-1598

National Wholesale Druggists' Association (NWDA)
1821 Michael Faraday Drive, Suite 400
Reston, Virginia 22090-5348

Pharmaceutical Manufacturers Association (PMA)
1100 Fifteenth Street N.W.
Washington, DC 20005

Uniform Code Council (UCC)
8163 Old Yankee Road, Suite J
Dayton, Ohio 45458

Trade Publications

ID Systems
Helmers Publishing Inc.
174 Concord Street
Peterborough, New Hampshire 03458

Automatic I.D. News
Advanstar Communications, Inc.
7500 Old Oak Boulevard
Cleveland, Ohio 44130

Index

About the Authors

Karen M. Longe is Marketing Manager, Healthcare for Zebra Technologies Corporation, a leading provider of bar code labeling solutions worldwide. In this capacity, Ms. Longe works with health care professionals and bar code manufacturers, distributors and software integrators to assure the development and dissemination of bar code printers and labels that satisfy healthcare market needs. Prior to joining Zebra, Ms. Longe was Manager of Program Planning and Development for the bar code program at the American Hospital Association. During her tenure at the AHA, she chaired the committee which developed the Health Industry Bar Code Provider Applications Standard. Ms. Longe is actively involved in standards development and education for the bar code industry in healthcare. She represents Zebra Technologies Corporation as its delegate to AIM USA and serves on the ScanTech Executive Committee. She is a frequent, international speaker about bar coding in healthcare and has written numerous articles on the subject. In 1989, Ms. Longe was awarded the prestigious Percival Award in recognition of her ongoing efforts in the bar code industry.

Lisa B. Brenner is Founder and President of Bright Ideas, a consulting firm that specializes in strategic marketing planning and communications development for health care clients and professional service businesses. Prior to founding the firm, Ms. Brenner directed a department in the development of corporate and marketing communications for the American Medical Association. She also served as Communications Manager at the American Hospital Association, where she collaborated with Ms. Longe in the development of bar code publications. Ms. Brenner holds a bachelor's degree in communications from Northwestern University. She has won numerous communications and design awards. She is a member of the American Society of Hospital Public Relations and Marketing and The Planning Forum.